Fit & Pregnant

The Pregnant Woman's Guide
to Exercise

by

Joan Marie Butler RNC, CNM

"The Menstrual Cycle Chart" is reprinted with permission from the Boston Women's Health Information Center. The chart was drawn by Peggy Clark and is found on page 256 of the 1992 edition of *The New Our Bodies, Ourselves*. New York: Simon and Schuster.

The *Recommendations for Exercise in Pregnancy and Postpartum* are used with the permission of the American College of Obstetricians and Gynecologists. They are found in Technical Bulletin No. 189, *Exercise During Pregnancy and the Postpartum Period*. ACOG, Washington, D.C. © 1994.

Library of Congress Cataloging-in-Publication Data

Butler, Joan Marie
    Fit & Pregnant : the pregnant woman's guide to exercise / Joan Marie Butler.
        p.   cm.
    Includes bibliographical references and index.
    ISBN 0-937921-55-6 : $16.00
    1. Pregnant women--Health and hygiene. 2. Exercise for women.
    3. Physical fitness for women. I. Title.
    RG558. 7 . B88 1995
    618.2 ' 4--dc20   95-32263
                                                                          CIP

Printed in the United States of America

TABLE OF CONTENTS

FOREWORDS

We are not far removed from the time when fitness was thought of as maintaining an ideal (or near ideal) body weight by following a variety of fad diets. The concept of exercise aiding the process of weight control was not a part of our consciousness. Likewise, the idea of cardiovascular and muscular fitness was secondary to weight. It was all part of the "looking good" that was, and in many ways still is, so entrenched in our society. From perfectly manicured lawns to meticulously coifed hair-dos to thin bodies, we spend an inordinate amount of time and energy making sure that everything about our lives looks good.

Recently, there has been a heightened interest in achieving and maintaining fitness. More than simply maintaining the right body size, fitness today implies a state of health that emphasizes body fat content, cardiovascular status, and muscular strength and tone. Recent publicity about the importance of low fat diets and aerobic exercise has captured the attention of many people. Medical research supports the belief that a longer and better life with fewer medical problems can be achieved through physical fitness. More people than ever are counting grams of fat, joining health clubs, and attending aerobic dance classes.

And now — comes the pregnant woman! There is no subject where science and myth are so intertwined than in pregnancy. Stop and think for a moment of some of the "old wives' tales," such sayings as "Don't raise your hands over your head ... it will make the cord wrap around the baby's neck," and "Don't lift anything during pregnancy."

Until recently, there has been little guidance for the fit woman during pregnancy. Each provider of health had his or her own ideas about exercise during pregnancy, and women heard many different opinions about what was healthy and what might be harmful. Fortunately, research in this vital area has provided us with a much clearer picture of the kinds and degrees of activities in which a pregnant woman can safely engage.

Fit and Pregnant provides a safe and effective guide to fitness for the woman experiencing a normal pregnancy. The author begins by noting the relationship between fitness and fertility. She then proceeds to outline the normal physical and emotional changes that occur during pregnancy and recommends some coping mechanisms and relief measures. Before describing specific exercises and fitness programs, she first carefully discusses the safety aspects of exercise in pregnancy. She takes into consideration the recommendations of such prestigious organizations as the American College of Obstetricians and Gynecologists and the American College of Sports Medicine. This is followed by a discussion of nutrition in an active pregnancy. The remainder of the book describes various ways that one can safely exercise throughout pregnancy and maintain fitness.

Drawing upon personal experience, the experiences of other active women, and medical research, Joan Butler has brought together in one volume, a "how to" approach to physical fitness during pregnancy. *Fit and Pregnant* will be a valuable asset to any woman who wishes to remain fit during pregnancy and after.

JAMES CAHILL M.D., F.A.C.O.G.
(Fellow, American College of OB/GYN)

Today, exercise is an integral part of many women's lives. They exercise competitively, for physical fitness, and for recreation. During pregnancy, these women are often eager to maintain an active lifestyle. Most can continue a moderate exercise program under the guidance of their physician or nurse-midwife.

This book is not a push to "do it all." Rather, it is a reference for exercise possibilities. It examines many popular physical activities such as running, swimming, cross-country skiing, cycling, aerobics, and weight training and provides the reader with specific advice on how to safely continue exercising while following the 1994 ACOG Guidelines for Exercise in Pregnancy. *Fit and Pregnant* even explores some pleasurable activities like canoeing and snowshoeing that you might want to add to your regime.

As health care providers, we see a pregnant woman monthly and eventually weekly. We need to take the time to discuss a woman's exercise program with her along with obstetric and medical history, lifestyle, social habits, occupation, and diet. Not every woman will be able to continue to exercise during her pregnancy. The prime concern is the safety of the fetus and the mother. Certain obstetrical complications (premature labor, premature rupture of membranes, incompetent cervix, hypertension, multiple gestation) may prohibit exercise during pregnancy.

The psychological benefits of exercise may be as important as the physical ones, especially in pregnancy. Many women view pregnancy as a source of added stress to an already full lifestyle with career pressures, family obligations, other children, school, etc. A program of exercise, even if it is several one-half hour sessions of aerobics, will give a woman a sense of accomplishment, motivation to stay fit, and an outlet for stress — this is "her" time.

Fit and Pregnant notes that pregnancy is a great time for couples to improve on nutrition and health habits. It encourages couples to use working out as a shared activity and common bonding time. I think that partners will also benefit from the educational material in this book. The partner may have fears and stresses regarding the pregnancy, birth, and addition to the home front. Some are not aware that moderate exercise is actually <u>beneficial</u> during pregnancy and not necessarily harmful.

There is a tremendous emphasis in our society on being perfect; the perfect physique being high on the list. Exercise clubs are popping up everywhere and many provide daycare and social activities. I have found in my practice that a tremendous source of anxiety for many pregnant women is weight gain, change in body image, and never returning to one's pre-pregnant weight. I recommend *Fit and Pregnant* as the treatment for these concerned women!

Joan Butler takes a realistic approach to the life demands during pregnancy and especially afterward. She offers many suggestions for activities that you can do right in the home and has practical advice on how to squeeze an exercise period into a busy schedule. *Fit and Pregnant* provides a compassionate and rational approach to the subject of exercise and pregnancy.

KRISTEN J. KRATZERT M.D., F.A.C.O.G.
(Fellow, American College of OB/GYN)

ACKNOWLEDGMENTS

I would like to thank the over one hundred women and their partners who shared their exercise experiences during their pregnancies and afterwards. Special thanks goes to Dick Mansfield who planted the idea for the project and skillfully edited the writing and format of the book. I wish to acknowledge the assistance, support and patience of my husband, John, and our son, Seth, whose arrival inspired the book.

The following people helped with their contributions, advice and encouragement.

Kathleen Aragon
Shannon Bliss
Phil Buckenmeyer, PhD
Martine Burat
Alane Butler
Patty Butler
Jennifer Bryant
James Cahill, M.D.
Kathryn Caiello, ACE Trainer
Gina Campoli
David Casieda, M.D.
Dan Chakin, ACE Trainer
Stephanie DeGirolamo
Patrick Dorr, M.D.
Penny Eagan
Cathleen Falge
Patty Ford
Susan Fritzell
Judy Geer
Lisa Glauber
Kathy Hahn
Mary Handley
Kristen Hartnett

Trish Heed
Carol Hillman-VanDyke
Sarah Huntington
Mary Janiszewski
Shelly, James and Sarah Kempton
Sara Kooperman, J.D.
Kristen Kratzert, M.D.
Cindy Lynch
Mary Martin
Eleanor Price McLees, CNM
Melissa Moody
Elizabeth Morgenthien
Janet Moskal
Sandy Palmer
Christine Pfitzinger
Lisa Powers
Genie Rotundo, RN, FACCE
Kathy Ruggeri
Wendy Sanders
Cydney and Marty Scarano
Sandra and Allen Spencer
Wendy Wilson
Judy Ziwicki-Gianforte

Introduction

More and more women today are exercising to stay fit. Women swell the ranks of walkers, cyclists, cross-country skiers, and runners and are responsible for much of the growth of activities such as aerobics, in-line skating, canoeing, and mountain biking. Some work out to control weight or to tone up; others do it just for recreation. A growing number of female athletes, from seven to seventy, train daily for competition in their chosen sport.

Do you fit into one of these exercise categories? Are you pregnant or considering becoming pregnant? If so, you are part of the new generation of women who are physically fit and athletic — and quite often wondering, along with their partners, just how to safely stay fit while pregnant.

Prior to the 1980's, physicians usually advised pregnant women to rest and avoid heavy exertion. In 1985, the American College of Obstetricians and Gynecologists (ACOG) established general guidelines for exercise during pregnancy. These guidelines were very broad and not applicable to the very fit woman. Fortunately, a new set of guidelines now calls for a more personalized approach to designing an exercise program. (See Chapter 3)

As a certified nurse-midwife and athletic woman, I am frequently asked about exercise and pregnancy. Patients, and their partners, are eager to work toward a healthy pregnancy and delivery. I find that many women share the common goal of staying fit during pregnancy and reaping the physiological as well as the psychological benefits of an exercise program.

I wrote this book to help women, at all levels of fitness, design a personal exercise program for their pregnancies. I look at pregnancy from the vantage point of the fit woman and start by discussing the effects of exercise on fertility. Then, I outline some of the physiological changes you can expect, review some of the basic exercise guidelines, and discuss nutrition. Throughout the book, I will be sharing with you some of the experiences from the pregnancies of fit women — world-class athletes to recreational exercisers. We will look together at a number of exercise activities that women use to stay fit during pregnancy. For each activity, I discuss some of the special body changes which occur during the course of a normal pregnancy. Finally, I cover postpartum exercise and how you and your newly expanded family can stay fit.

The material and guidance I share with you is from current research on the topic and my fifteen years of working with pregnant women. My own exercise program before, during, and after pregnancy, gave me insight and inspiration as did the experiences of other active women I interviewed.

Each pregnancy is special and each exercise program will be unique. You should work closely with your nurse-midwife or physician in personalizing your own program to be Fit and Pregnant.

1

EXERCISE AND FERTILITY

Since you are reading this book, I suspect that you are a woman who exercises and are either pregnant, or planning to become pregnant. That's great! As you will see in the chapters ahead, exercise is an important component of a healthy pregnancy. What we are going to do in this first chapter is to look at how exercise, particularly when it is at an intense level, may affect your ability to conceive. Let's start by discussing menstrual cycles.

MENSTRUAL CYCLES

Janet is a 43 year old mother of four and a runner. Back before her first child, she noticed, while training for a marathon, a change in her menstrual cycles when she increased her running mileage from 25 to 40 to 50 miles a week. Her periods were further apart and she missed one period. Though her weight stayed the same, it took six months for her cycles to return to normal after the marathon. She conceived her first baby four months later. With her subsequent pregnancies, she cut back her mileage during the times she was trying to get pregnant.

Ann, a 32 year old triathlete, noticed that during the summer months she occasionally missed one or two periods. She typically spent most summers training more seriously and racing two or three weekends a month. Ann is a small muscular woman whose weight would drop three or four pounds during this time of intense athletic activity. Her cycles were normal during the winter months.

To better understand the exercise-related changes in Janet's and Ann's menstrual cycles, let's first take a look at how our reproductive cycles normally work. A normal menstrual cycle is between 20 and 40 days. To determine the interval between your periods, count from the first day of one period to the first day of your next period. If you have a 28 day cycle, the first half of the cycle, days 1 through 14, is called the follicular phase. The second half, days 14 to 28 is the luteal phase.

Your hypothalamus and pituitary glands, located in the brain, send messages through hormones to your ovaries and uterus. The hypothalamus gland signals the pituitary gland to release follicle stimulating hormone (FSH). In turn, FSH stimulates your ovaries to develop follicles — immature eggs. These follicles then release the hormone estrogen which causes the lining of the uterus to become thicker in preparation for pregnancy. As the estrogen levels rise, luteinizing hormone (LH) and FSH rise to peak levels. This surge in hormones releases a mature egg from the ovary — causing ovulation. Pregnancy can occur if a sperm joins the egg and fertilization takes place. For the next two weeks, the luteal phase of the cycle, the hormone progesterone further prepares the lining of the uterus for implantation of the fertilized egg. If pregnancy does not occur, the progesterone level drops and bleeding begins around day 28. The bleeding continues for three to seven days.

Not all women fit this 28-day cycle, though most have fairly regular menstrual cycles. The interval from menstruation to ovulation can vary, but the time between ovulation and menstruation is the most consistent for all of us and is usually 14 days. It is possible to have a period without ovulation and vice versa, but usually amenorrhea — missing periods — signals a disruption in ovulation. If you are not ovulating, you cannot conceive.

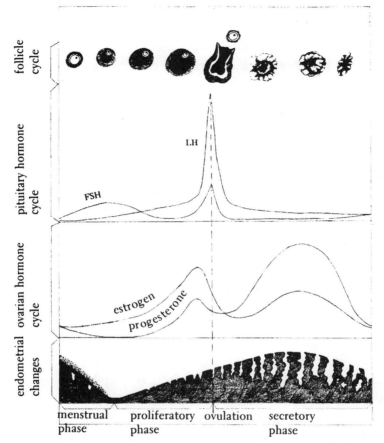

The menstrual cycle: the relationship between follicle development, hormone cycles, and endometrial (uterine lining) buildup and disintegration. The cervical mucus gets progressively wetter from the menstrual phase to ovulation, then becomes drier during the secretory phase.   **Peggy Clark**

MENSTRUAL IRREGULARITIES

Recent research has helped us to understand some of the effects of exercise on our menstrual cycles, but there is still much that we do not understand. From what we do know, we recognize that there are many causes of irregular cycles. Basically, irregular cycles are due to a disruption in how the hypothalamus communicates with the pituitary gland, ovaries, and uterus. This may result in amenorrhea (absence of menstrual periods), oligomenorrhea (infrequent periods), or a disturbance in the luteal phase of the cycle.

How does exercise affect your menstrual cycles? Let's use running as an example. When you run at high intensity, doing such things as speedwork, competing, or running more than 30 miles a week, you cause a rise in beta-endorphins. (Suddenly increasing your mileage can have the same effect.) These "feel good" hormones give you a "runner's high," but they also can suppress the release of gonadotropins (FSH and LH) from the pituitary gland. Similarly, vigorous running releases cortisol (a "stress" hormone) from the adrenal glands. High cortisol levels also interfere with the release of FSH and LH. When this happens, ovulation does not occur and menstruation ceases.

Researchers (Heltland et al. 1993) who examined the menstrual cycles of 205 runners, found that elite runners who ran up to 80 miles a week were at greatest risk for developing amenorrhea. The runners who developed amenorrhea had lower levels of estrogen and a drop in their bone density. Low estrogen levels, which also occur in menopause, put these runners at risk for stress fractures and osteoporosis (bone-thinning).

Body fat and body weight also play a role in menstrual irregularities but perhaps not as significant as we once thought. Our bodies need a certain percentage of body fat to maintain our reproductive cycles and ultimately to support pregnancy and lactation. If we reduce these energy stores, we can in turn disrupt our menstrual cycles. Athletic amenorrhea is more common in individual competitive sports like running, gymnastics, ballet and figure skating where a slim body is desirable. Pressure to excel plus the emphasis on low body weight can put these women at risk.

Besides body fat and the physical stress of exercise, psychological stress seems to play a role in menstrual irregularities. Under stress, the adrenal glands release cortisol, which, as mentioned above, is known to interfere with the release of FSH and LH. A classic study in 1965 (Shanan et al., 1965) examined 65 young

American women who went to live in Israel for a year. Twenty-two percent of them temporarily stopped menstruating while abroad. These women had higher cortisol levels probably due to the stress and anxiety of being away from home and living in a foreign country. Intense exercise can be psychologically, as well as physically stressful for some athletic women and elevate cortisol levels. This biological response to stress appears to prepare the body for challenge and directs energy away from reproduction.

"FEMALE ATHLETIC TRIAD"

"Female athletic triad" refers to the relationship of three medical disorders — disordered eating, amenorrhea, and osteoporosis. Current research has examined the prevalence and potential risks associated with these collective disorders. The term "triad" means that the three problems are often seen together and are related.

Competitive female athletes, especially runners, gymnasts, ballet dancers, and figure skaters feel pressure to maintain a certain body weight for aesthetics and improved performance. This "striving for thinness" may lead to food restrictions, fasting, binging (overeating), or purging (vomiting and laxative abuse). The extreme end of this is anorexia nervosa when body weight drops below 15% of normal. Recurrent episodes of binge eating followed by purging is called bulimia. Reduced body weight or fat can lead to amenorrhea, or oligomenorrhea (infrequent periods) or luteal phase defects. As mentioned before, luteal phase suppression occurs when there is inadequate progesterone in the second half of your menstrual cycle. These athletes place themselves at particular risk for the athletic triad.

Low levels of the reproductive hormones — estrogen and progesterone — can cause osteoporosis — premature bone loss and inadequate bone formation. We usually gain our peak bone mass by age eighteen. For the next twelve years or so, we have the potential to gain bone mass. Studies have shown that some young athletes with amenorrhea may have decreased bone mineral density. Thinner, less dense bone presents a greater risk for stress fractures and premature osteoporotic fractures.

It is not clear just how prevalent the athletic triad is. One reason is that athletes affected by this problem may deny or hide the symptoms. Another reason is that the study results are varied: disordered eating patterns in female athletes may be between 15% to 62% (Rosen and Hough 1988; Rosen et al. 1986) and the incidence of amenorrhea between 3.4% and 66%(Otis 1992; Shangold 1988). There is no evidence to show what the incidence of osteoporosis may be. Treatment for the problem of female athletic triad may require medical, psychological and nutritional intervention. Prevention and education are also important. Females in "at risk" sports need to develop safe training techniques as well as positive and realistic body images and proper nutritional guidance.

TOO MUCH OF A GOOD THING?

There is no specific amount of weight loss, body fat percentage, exercise or stress level that will cause menstrual changes for all women. For example, Roxanne is a runner who averages 40 miles a week. While training for marathons, she increases this to 60 to 70 miles. Normally her menstrual cycles are 28 days apart but during the marathon season they are every 22 to 23 days. In contrast, Gail and Alisa, both competitive runners, average 80 to 100 miles a week and have regular menstrual cycles. In fact, Alisa, whose body fat is approximately 9%, (most women average 22%) conceived shortly after a vigorous racing season.

Remember, each of us reacts differently to emotional stress. Stress is a part of everyday life, but how we cope is individual. What is stressful to one person may not cause the same reaction in someone else. Our own biology, personality and experience seem to dictate how vulnerable we are to stress. Now, before pregnancy, is a good time to take a look at how you handle stress in your life. The demands of parenting will certainly introduce you to all kinds of new sources of stress. If you find yourself "addicted" to exercise, you need to weigh how much exercise actually reduces stress and how much the compulsion to exercise puts more pressure on you. It is important to find that comfortable middle ground where you reap the rewards, both physical and psychological, of an exercise program but are not driven solely by the goals of exercise.

CAN I GET PREGNANT?

If you are missing periods it is likely that you are not ovulating and will not be able to get pregnant. It is important that the underlying cause of your amenorrhea be determined by a gynecological exam and special tests. You can usually reverse infertility caused by exercise once you cut back on the duration or intensity of your exercise program or, if you are too thin, by gaining weight. If you need to gain weight, now is a good time to improve your eating habits and adopt a healthy diet that is rich in calcium before conception (See Chapter 4). Depending on your clinical evaluation you may need to take hormones to stimulate ovulation.

If you are trying to conceive, take a look at your current exercise program. What are your fitness goals? How often are you exercising and at what intensity? Are you training for competition or exercising for fun and fitness? Your program should include aerobic activity (running, cycling, aerobics class, walking) for at least 20 minutes 3 to 5 times a week. Concentrate on building muscle strength, aerobic endurance, and overall stamina. Blend weight-bearing activities like running and aerobics with non-impact sports (swimming, cycling). If you are out of shape, begin with low impact sports such as walking, and start slowly.

Visit your health care provider for a physical and health assessment before trying to get pregnant. If you are a competitive athlete, discuss how your pregnancy plans will fit into your "off season" of training. Review your obstetric and medical history as well as diet and exercise program. Talk about your lifestyle, the work you do, and the type of environment you live in (urban, rural, etc.). Start thinking about the type of practitioner from whom you would like to receive your obstetric care — an obstetrician/gynecologist, a family practitioner or certified nurse-midwife. It is important to find a practitioner who is knowledgeable about exercise during pregnancy. Consider your options for place of birth. Do you want to use a hospital labor and delivery room, birthing rooms within the hospital, or a free-standing birth center? Be sure to talk to other women about their pregnancy experiences. After considering all these issues, make a decision that fits you and your partner's needs for one of life's most joyous ventures.

WHAT OTHERS SAY

Here are some pre-pregnancy comments from active women I interviewed.

"I generally stayed healthy and consumed no alcohol when I was trying to get pregnant."

"I was undergoing infertility treatment, so I moderated my exercise and tried to eat better."

"I was training for a diving competition when I got pregnant on our honeymoon."

"My pregnancy was not planned, so I did not cut back on my training schedule." (A competitive runner with a 5k personal record of 16:07.)

"I wished I had gotten in better shape before pregnancy. I gained 10 pounds over the winter and bad weather forced me to reduce my running."

"I had broken my foot so we decided to have children. I went from peak racing form (5k personal record 15:12) to a foot in a cast and trying to get pregnant. It only took us one month to conceive."

"Both of my pregnancies occurred while running nearly 100 miles a week." (A competitive runner)

"I had a complete physical and started taking vitamins and eliminated all alcohol. We conceived two months later."

2

YOUR CHANGING BODY

Change is what pregnancy is all about. You will be struck at times during your pregnancy by the dramatic and sometimes overwhelming changes occurring in your body. It can be startling to suddenly look down and see a moving swollen "ball" where there once was a waistline. This kind of change is obvious, but other changes are subtle. Changes are both physical and emotional.

For some women, pregnancy is a time when they feel their best and have a sense of inner calm and untapped energy. Others, less fortunate, are plagued by persistent nausea, heartburn, or backache. The changes initiated by pregnancy start soon after conception, continue right up to delivery and postpartum, and call for you to make both mental and physical adaptations.

The first adaptation you'll face is the reality of being pregnant and all that it means. For many, the response to the news of pregnancy, whether it was planned or not, is one of ambivalence. This is quite normal. You will be trying to imagine the journey ahead, the new demands and role changes, and the tremendous physical changes that will occur. Talking about these mixed feelings (joy, fear, anxiety) and honestly accepting the mixture of emotions as "normal" seems to help most women. If you are active, you may focus more on the physical aspects of pregnancy and on your changing body. Let's look at some of the physical changes you will face.

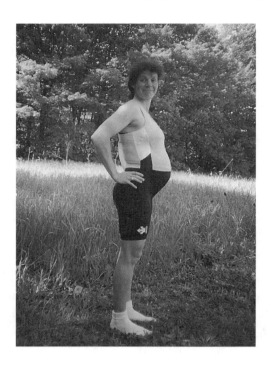

For some women, pregnancy is a time when they feel their best.

PHYSIOLOGICAL CHANGES

FIRST TRIMESTER
Fatigue

Fatigue is often one of the early signs of pregnancy. If you are used to having a lot of energy and going out and exercising each day, you may be surprised by this early sign. Fatigue is often described as an all-consuming feeling of being tired and without energy — and it seems to arrive regardless of sleep. A combination of factors, the most important being the tremendous hormone changes you are undergoing and the metabolic demands of the growing fetus, cause fatigue.

Active women must create a balance between exercise and rest. There will be days when your body is telling you to cut back on exercise — so do it. Take short breaks or take an exercise day off to help you get through this phase. Your impulse may be to fight the fatigue and "gut it out" — doing more or forcing yourself to complete a preset goal. But this is the time to surrender, listen to your body, and realize that by the end of the third month, the veil of fatigue will probably begin to lift.

Breast Changes

The hormones of pregnancy, estrogen and progesterone, are responsible for breast changes throughout pregnancy. In the first few months your breasts may be tender and swollen. The nipples may become very sensitive to touch or to the friction from bras or clothing. You can do several things to help alleviate this problem.

Additional breast support which controls breast motion and allows for evaporation of moisture will help you feel more comfortable. It may also help to avoid synthetic fabrics. If you run or do aerobics, try a supportive cotton bra with wide adjustable straps or a sports bra. One elite runner, during her first pregnancy, told me that she wore two bras for added support.

If you are a runner or "stair climber," a temporary change to swimming or cycling — sports which are less jarring — will probably help. Though your breasts continue to enlarge throughout pregnancy, the tenderness tends to abate so you will eventually be able to resume your usual exercises. Later in pregnancy, however, your breasts may begin to leak. The hormone prolactin causes this early milk secretion in preparation for lactation. Wear nursing pads or cut a panty liner to fit the inside of the bra during exercise to solve this problem.

Nausea

"Morning sickness" — waves of queasiness which can hit anytime or any place — is one of the classic trademarks of pregnancy. For me, the smell of sweaty polypropylene clothing would trigger waves of flu-like feelings. I banned my husband's running top from the house for the first three months of my pregnancy. Mary, a competitive cyclist, "never thought (because she is healthy and an athlete) she would feel so ill." Her nausea and dry heaves occurred day and night during her first trimester.

Nausea commonly occurs in over half of all pregnancies. A combination of hormonal changes, a slowed digestive system, the growing uterus, and emotional factors are all causes. The symptoms tend to be worse when your stomach is empty or when you are fatigued so the key to combating it lies in those two areas.

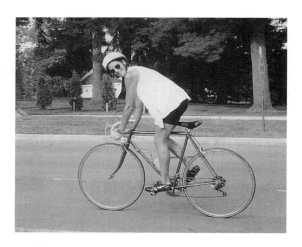

An outdoor activity like cycling may offer relief from nausea.

There are numerous relief measures. Some common remedies include these: eat small frequent meals, maintain a high protein and complex carbohydrate diet, and take vitamin B6 supplements. Some women have found relief using TravelBands,™ SeaBands,™ or BioBands™ which are applied to the wrists and put pressure on the inner wrist. This is a form of accupressure which may reduce the sensation of nausea. These are available through pharmacies and some travel bureaus and catalogs. Morning Sickness: All Day and All Night is a video which offers advice on the subject. See Resource Section for more information.

Nausea may interfere with your desire to exercise. It also may force you to change the timing of your workouts. For example, if you normally exercise at the end of the day when you may be tired and hungry, consider a morning or middle of the day workout. An Olympic champion runner and mother of two said that she avoided nausea by running first thing in the morning and then eating a substantial breakfast. If you are normally an indoor exerciser, try some fresh air — pursuing an outdoor activity such as running, cycling, or skiing may offer some relief from nausea.

Frequent Urination

Early in pregnancy, as the uterus grows, pressure is exerted on the bladder. The need to urinate will often come during the night (nocturia) or during exercise when you place more pressure on your bladder, especially during running or aerobics. Just plan to empty your bladder before your workout and if needed, during physical activity. Don't, by any means, restrict fluid intake. During your pregnancy, you should drink at least eight glasses of water a day. Hydrate before exercise and keep a water bottle handy. Drinking fluids helps you keep cool during a workout. Water bottles are handy. I recommend that you drink just water — avoid the sports drinks until after the pregnancy.

SECOND TRIMESTER

During the second trimester (months four, five and six), your body changes will become more apparent. You will feel more comfortable in looser fitting clothing and will want to accommodate your expanding waistline with elastic waistlines or loose oversized shirts. I will discuss specific workout wear for pregnancy and specific sports in future chapters.

Backache

Low back pain occurs to some extent in most pregnancies. The combination of weight gain and the enlarging uterus alters your center of gravity. You will tend to compensate by drawing your shoulders back and walking with a sway back. This curvature of the lower back is what causes the aching sensation of muscle strain. Women who have relatively strong abdominal muscles are able to give support to the growing uterus and have less muscle strain in the back — so get those abdominals in shape before pregnancy!

Backache can also be a sign of overuse (doing too much exercise) or excessive bending and lifting. Learn how to lift now. Proper body mechanics are important. If you bend at the knees, and not at the waist, and spread your feet apart with one foot slightly in front of the other, you will help save your back. Following pregnancy, when you're lifting a small child and carrying all sorts of baby equipment, you'll be glad that you learned to lift properly.

Heartburn and indigestion

The hormones estrogen and progesterone tend to relax the smooth muscle in the gastrointestinal tract which in turn slows down the digestive process. Bloating and indigestion can develop as food sits in the digestive tract. Some women experience heartburn near the end of the second trimester and into the third trimester. Heartburn, or regurgitation of gastric contents, is caused by a relaxation of the cardiac sphincter of the stomach and displacement and compression of the stomach by the uterus, allowing stomach acid to leave the stomach and enter the esophagus.

There are a number of steps you can take which may provide relief. Eat small, frequent meals, thus avoiding over-distention of the stomach; avoid spicy and fried foods or carbonated drinks; and sleep with your head slightly elevated (an extra pillow may help). Use good posture and body alignment to prevent further pressure on the stomach. Exercise several hours after a meal and wear loose non-restrictive clothing around the abdomen or waist.

Constipation and hemorrhoids

As just mentioned, pregnancy hormones, specifically progesterone, slow down the digestive process. The growing uterus causes displacement and compression of the bowel. If you take separate iron supplements for anemia (low iron levels), you may be plagued by constipation. If you had problems with constipation before, pregnancy will increase these problems.

Constipation can contribute to the development of hemorrhoids. Pressure from the growing uterus and straining when having a bowel movement cause dilation of the hemorrhoidal tissue (rectal veins). Diet is an important prevention for both constipation and hemorrhoids. Drinking eight to ten glasses of water a day and eating foods which provide roughage, bulk, and natural fiber is important (see Chapter 4 — Nutrition). Take stool softeners only if advised by your health care provider.

You can relieve the discomfort of hemorrhoids by taking warm tub baths or by applying witch hazel compresses, ice packs, or local analgesic ointments. You can help relieve pressure to the area by lying down with your legs raised. Avoid cycling for long periods or weight training with the Valsalva maneuver (holding your breath and straining) because these activities put more pressure on the dilated veins.

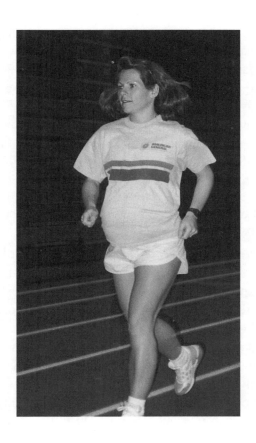

Your running gait may change as your pregnancy advances.

Ligament and joint changes

During pregnancy, the hormone relaxin is being released. Relaxin helps loosen joints and connective tissue to accommodate the growing uterus and to help in delivery through the birth canal. For some women this can be a very subtle change, and for others, the feeling of "shifting bones" in the pelvic region is more dramatic. If you continue to run, you are likely to be more aware of these changes. Your running gait may change, and because your entire musculoskeletal system is softening, injury may occur.

It happened to me. I developed a tendinitis of the ankle region at about sixteen weeks into my pregnancy. At the time, I was surprised at the sudden onset of the injury, but now I realize that it was probably due to a combination of factors: connective tissue changes, change in my running gait, and the additional few pounds of weight. I was able to cycle and swim for a few weeks and then started Stairmaster‰ workouts. I returned to running when all pain was gone and bought a new pair of running shoes which were softer and provided more support.

Proper warm up and stretching is essential to any workout in pregnancy (See Chapter 5). You need to listen to early warning signs, especially pain during or after a workout. This is not the time to run through or ignore a body signal.

THIRD TRIMESTER

Varicosities

The development of varicosities in the leg or vulvar area during pregnancy is more apt to occur if there is a family history or genetic predisposition. Rapid weight gain or tight restrictive clothing contributes to the problem. Also, progesterone, one of pregnancy's hormones, plays a role by causing the relaxation of the vein walls and the surrounding smooth muscles. Further pressure is placed on the pelvic veins by the expanded blood volume and the weight of the growing uterus.

If you have been physically active prior to pregnancy, you may be less apt to develop varicose veins. During pregnancy, exercise such as running and aerobics will help to improve circulation in the pelvic region and legs. If painful varicosities should develop, consider shortening an exercise routine or changing to another form of activity (less weight bearing). Kathy, a thirty-two year old mother of three, developed varicosities during her third pregnancy. When the varices became uncomfortable during aerobic workouts, she shortened her routine and supplemented it by swimming.

You can obtain some relief by elevating your legs periodically during the day or by wearing supportive hose. You can provide support to the vulvar varices by wearing two snugly placed sanitary pads with a sanitary belt.

Swelling

Most women will develop some mild swelling of the ankles or feet at some time during the pregnancy. Your growing uterus puts pressure on the blood vessels which return fluid from the legs. Restrictive clothing around the ankles, legs, or pelvic area impedes circulation and prolonged standing causes swelling in your legs and ankles. Swelling is usually most noticeable at the end of the day or in warm weather.

Adequate hydration (eight to ten glasses of liquid a day) helps the kidneys to work more effectively and reduces swelling. You can help by elevating your legs periodically, by avoiding crossing your legs, and by wearing comfortable supportive shoes, especially when exercising. I found that in the last few weeks of pregnancy, I was more comfortable running in a shoe with flexible uppers and more cushioning in the sole.

Braxton Hicks Contractions

Braxton Hicks contractions (first observed by J. Braxton Hicks in the 19th century) usually begin sometime after the twentieth week of pregnancy. They are a painless tightening of the muscles in the uterus and become more frequent in the last month. Braxton Hicks differ from labor contractions because they are sporadic and non-rhythmic. Sometimes it is difficult to distinguish between Braxton Hicks contractions and premature labor or labor. If they occur more than four in an hour or with any kind of pain, you should notify your health care provider.

You can think of Braxton Hicks contractions as a "warm-up" session for labor. Changing your position or activity may stop the tightening of the uterine muscles. If they occur during exercise, stop or slow down and concentrate on slow deep breathing. This is an opportunity to listen to the signals your body is sending and "tune in." Runners may experience these tightenings while running. Slowing down or walking for a few minutes should help.

YOUR CHANGING BODY — YOUR CHANGING SELF

As you can see, your body will be changing tremendously during the next nine months. Carrying a child and giving birth is probably one of the most powerful experiences we will have in our lives. It is a period of both tremendous physical and emotional transformation — as we begin to integrate ourselves into the upcoming role of caretaker and parent. Our sense of self begins to change as our bodies change. There are new sensations, limitations, and opportunities for self awareness. Part of this emotional adjustment is body image. Our once familiar "self" suddenly encounters the "pregnant self," and for some women these images can create a conflict.

Body Image

Our society places heavy emphasis on the "ideal" female body — the firm, trim figure — and this ideal frequently compels many women to exercise. Some of you have worked hard through diet and exercise to get to this ideal state, or at least close to it. Now you are pregnant, and even if anticipated and met with joy, your pregnancy brings on the body changes we just discussed, and such changes may be at odds with your vision.

It is easy to think that you will maintain control with diet and more exercise — the same way you did before you were pregnant. You hope that continued exercise will be your salvation to restore you to your slim state after nine months of expansion. Many women fear getting bigger and then staying that way after the baby.

Our culture offers limited support on this topic. The "ideal" female image is in direct contrast to the basic biology of being female. If you allow yourself to accept this image, pregnancy may become a frustrating barrier to staying trim, fit, and athletic.

A NOTE TO FATHERS

Fathers-to-be play a significant role in a woman's feelings about herself in pregnancy. As a "partner in reproduction," you also need to learn as much as you can about the physical as well as emotional changes of pregnancy. Patience and understanding are the key words during the next nine months. Listen to your partner's concerns and appreciate the tremendous responsibility she is assuming in nurturing the baby's growth. As the most significant person in her life, you need to offer words of encouragement and support. I can remember asking my husband if I looked "big" in my eighth month. (I was feeling huge and didn't think I could possibly get any bigger.) His response was, "You look great!" At those critical moments when her self-esteem is teetering, she will need some ego boosting.

Fathers-to-be are also going through a change in identity. You are essentially on the outside of the construction site, but your concerns may be very similar. You will find yourself concerned about the health of the developing fetus and your partner, apprehensive about labor and delivery as well as the impact of parenthood and lifestyle changes. Talking about all these concerns will help you both get through the next nine months. Partners can even adopt a "pregnant status." Why not strive for a healthier diet, avoid unhealthy habits, and spend time exercising together? A teamwork approach can start now and blossom during parenthood.

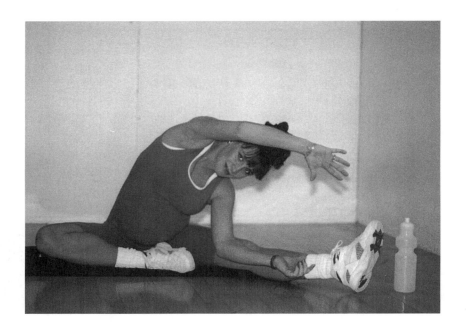

Exercise can build self-confidence as your body changes.

Emotional Passage

The early signs of pregnancy, the breast tenderness, nausea, or fatigue, signal the mysterious beginnings of new life. What follows are more changes. Some are not so subtle. Vigorous kicking or lower backache can be the ever constant reminders of your connection to the growing fetus inside. It is inevitable that conflicts will develop between your needs (e.g., sleep, back relief) and the needs of the fetus.

Exercise and body awareness can help calm the conflicts and nurture this connection. Women who engage in regular exercise are well attuned to their body and the signals that it sends. Physical activity or athletic competition provides us an opportunity to listen to the signals our body might be sending that warn about overtraining or pain, or about possible injury. This increased body awareness may help you better cope with the variety of physiological changes that you will encounter in your pregnancy.

Bridging The Gap

I encourage women to learn as much as possible about their growing, changing bodies. This knowledge will help you gain a sense of trust in your body as it adapts to pregnancy. Libraries and bookstores are brimming with books on the topic. Share this information with your partner. Talk about all your sensations and changes. Talk with other women, especially other pregnant women and new mothers. Attend childbirth preparation classes with your partner for the opportunity to learn more about your pregnancy and to be around other couples like yourselves. Staying physically active and enjoying the benefits of exercise will help you bridge the gap and enjoy cooperating with your body for the next nine months.

WHAT OTHERS SAY

Here are some comments from women like yourselves who exercised during their pregnancies:

"Exercise allowed me to deal with my changing body more easily. I felt like I could control one aspect of my life."

" I felt stronger and more confident about my pregnancy because of exercise."

"Exercise helped my physical and emotional upkeep."

"It (exercise) gave me emotional strength in dealing with the hormonal mood swings."

"I felt a little more in control of my body which seemed so out of my control."

"Exercise really lifted my spirits and helped me feel positive about getting larger."

"Exercise allowed me to clear my head."

"Exercise is so much a part of my daily routine that I would have had a hard time emotionally if I had quit altogether."

"I felt strong. I had more stamina and endurance and a positive attitude."

Here are some comments from their partners:

"Don't discourage your wife from exercising ... they need it for their mental well-being."

"Encourage exercise but also make sure they (pregnant women) cooperate with what their bodies' are telling them."

"I encouraged her to do whatever made her feel good."

"I was happy that my wife continued her exercise program because I could see the benefits she gained from it, but I was concerned that she not overdue it."

The exercise goals of pregnancy are to maintain a safe level of fitness for you and your unborn baby. With these goals, an exercise program can help improve your body image and provide a sense of well being and self confidence as your body changes.

3

SAFETY FIRST — EXERCISE GUIDELINES

Today, exercise has become an integral part of many women's lives. In the sixties and seventies, Ken Cooper, Jim Fixx, Jane Fonda, and others espoused the benefits of regular aerobic exercise to a receptive audience. As a result, the "fitness" business boomed. Health clubs, fitness videos, home exercise equipment, and workout attire now flood the market place. The expansion of women's sports at both the scholastic and collegiate levels fosters a lifelong continuation of physical activity for many women. Most of our grandmothers led sedentary lives, but women today are creating a legacy of health and fitness for future generations.

If you exercise regularly, you have likely discovered the physical, psychological as well as social benefits of physical activity. There are different rewards for each of us. We're out there running, cycling, or swimming to maintain cardiovascular fitness, to strengthen our bones and muscles, to control weight, and to seek mental relaxation. We like the "mental high" we feel after an invigorating run or aerobics class -- the release of endorphins, the hormones which help to control pain and elevate our moods. Besides this sense of well being, we've found that staying fit can be a lot of fun. Lasting friendships are formed while circling the track, cycling around the countryside, or turning laps in a pool. Many active couples share the same love and enthusiasm for a particular sport or activity.

With the news of your pregnancy, all these "payoffs" of exercise that you have been enjoying need not cease. Yet, it is common for both you and your partner to wonder, "What exercise is safe for the next nine months?" When I first learned of my pregnancy, I was both thrilled and concerned — I wanted to know everything about my pregnancy, and, like other physically active women, I was eager to know how exercise might fit into the journey ahead. Let me share some of the things I learned.

The first thing I learned is that although the benefits of a regular exercise program are well established for both men and women; unfortunately, the proof of such benefits aren't as clear for pregnant women. But, the one thing that is clear is that there is no evidence to suggest that you should stop exercising just because you are pregnant.

While there have been a lot of studies addressing exercise and pregnancy, most of the early work was done with pregnant animals, raising questions about just how valid the findings were for pregnant women. Even some current studies have questionable results due to design flaws. But in recent years, because of the growing interest in exercise and pregnancy, new studies are focusing on how both the baby and the mother adapt to exercise. In reviewing the latest studies, it is evident that there is no need to automatically cease exercising during your pregnancy.

No, pregnancy is not an excuse to "gestate" and become a couch potato, but neither is it a time to start up a strenuous sport or train for the Olympics. As we shall see, the majority of you can continue to do most types of activities, while adjusting to your body's changes over the next nine months. It is important that you honestly assess your own level of fitness and design an exercise plan with the guidance of your health care provider. There are some recently-released guidelines that can help you both tailor a program for your pregnancy.

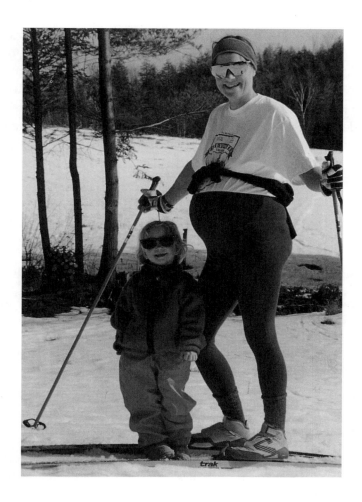

There is no evidence to suggest that you should
stop exercising just because you are pregnant.

EXERCISE AND PREGNANCY GUIDELINES

Until 1985, there were no written guidelines for exercise in
pregnancy. The American College of Obstetricians and Gynecologists (ACOG) published a bulletin in May of 1985, entitled "Exercise During Pregnancy and the Postnatal Period." This educational
bulletin addressed a broad section of the population and was to be
used as a guide for health care providers.

These early guidelines had some strict limitations. The bulletin advised women to keep their heart rate at 140 beats per minute and not engage in strenuous exercise for more than fifteen minutes. Adhering to those parameters, a well- conditioned woman would hardly be breaking into a sweat. Unfortunately, health care providers relied heavily on this bulletin and given the medical-legal atmosphere, were reluctant to deviate from the prescribed recommendations, even for very fit women.

In February 1994, ACOG modified these guidelines based on more current research which examines a woman's physiological adaptations to exercise in pregnancy and the effects on the fetus.

ACOG GUIDELINES
Recommendations for Exercise in Pregnancy and Postpartum

There are no data in humans to indicate that pregnant women should limit exercise intensity and lower target heart rates because of potential adverse effects. For women who do not have any additional risk factors for adverse maternal or perinatal outcome, the following recommendations may be made:

During pregnancy, women can continue to exercise and derive health benefits even from mild-to-moderate exercise routines. Regular exercise (at least three times per week) is preferable to intermittent activity.

Women should avoid exercise in the supine position [lying on the back] after the first trimester. Such a position is associated with decreased cardiac output in most pregnant women; because the remaining cardiac output will be preferentially distributed away from splanchnic beds [the gut area] (including the uterus) during vigorous exercise, such regimes are best avoided during pregnancy. Prolonged periods of motionless standing should also be avoided.

Women should be aware of the decreased oxygen available for aerobic exercise during pregnancy. They should be encouraged to modify the intensity of their exercise according to maternal symptoms. Pregnant women should stop exercising when fatigued and not exercise to exhaustion. Weight-bearing exercises may under some circumstances be continued at intensities similar to those prior to pregnancy throughout pregnancy. Non-weight bearing exercises such as cycling or swimming will minimize the risk of injury and facilitate the continuation of exercise during pregnancy.

Morphologic changes in pregnancy should serve as a relative contraindication to types of exercise in which loss of balance could be detrimental to maternal or fetal well-being, especially in the third trimester. Further, any type of exercise involving the potential for even mild abdominal trauma should be avoided.

Pregnancy requires an additional 300 kcal/d in order to maintain metabolic homeostasis. Thus, women who exercise during pregnancy should be particularly careful to ensure an adequate diet.

Pregnant women who exercise in the first trimester should augment heat dissipation by ensuring adequate hydration, appropriate clothing, and optimal environmental surroundings during exercise.

Many of the physiologic and morphologic changes of pregnancy persist 4-6 weeks postpartum. Thus, prepregnancy exercise routines should be resumed gradually based on a woman's physical capability.

Contraindications to Exercise

The aforementioned recommendations are intended for women who do not have any additional risk factors for adverse maternal or perinatal outcome. A number of medical and obstetric conditions may lead the obstetrician to recommend modifications of these principles. The following conditions should be considered contraindications to exercise during pregnancy:

Pregnancy-induced hypertension
Preterm rupture of membranes
Preterm labor during the prior or current pregnancy or both
Incompetent cervix/cerclage
Persistent second — or third — trimester bleeding
Intrauterine growth retardation
Multiple gestation

In addition, women with certain other medical or obstetric conditions, including chronic hypertension or active thyroid, cardiac, vascular, or pulmonary disease, should be evaluated carefully in order to determine whether an exercise program is appropriate.

Reprinted with permission from the American College of Obstetricians and Gynecologists. Exercise During Pregnancy and the Postpartum Period. Technical Bulletin No 189, ACOG, Washington, DC © 1994.

The American College of Sports Medicine (ACSM) has also voiced their opinion on exercise and pregnancy. The ACSM published a review of recent investigations on the topic. (McMurray et al. 1993). In this review they also looked at the maternal and fetal responses to exercise in addition to examining animal research models as well as pregnancy and physical conditioning. The data examined by the ACSM basically comes up with the same conclusions as ACOG. A pregnant woman can exercise safely during her pregnancy as long as she is aware of her body temperature (avoid overheating) and listens to her body signals (e.g., pain, fatigue). The ACSM echoes the importance of developing an exercise program in consultation with your health care provider.

These new guidelines allow for a more individualized approach to exercise and encourage health care providers to help a woman develop an exercise program based on her current level of fitness and the health of her pregnancy. Let's take a look at how your body adapts to exercise during pregnancy and some of the areas of concern for you and your baby.

BODY CHANGES AND EXERCISE

Pregnancy, as you learned in the last chapter, causes tremendous changes in your body. Your blood volume, cardiac output (amount of blood your heart pumps with each beat), and resting pulse all increase to help support the growing needs of the fetus as well as your own increase in size. This is all happening while you are resting and not even exercising. What happens when you start to run or cross-country ski?

When you exercise, you will become aware of some of the changes occurring in your heart and lungs due to pregnancy. You most likely will feel breathless or short of breath as you begin to exercise because your growing uterus pushes your diaphragm upward which reduces the space for your lungs to expand. The hormones of pregnancy also reduce your tolerance to carbon dioxide, which in turn, causes a state of hyperventilation both at rest and with exercise. An Olympic runner and mother of two reported, "I was breathing like an ox at the beginning of runs."

Despite this shortness of breath, your body can adapt to moderate levels of exercise, especially if you are physically fit before becoming pregnant. As you might expect, your exercise performance will decline as your pregnancy advances. This seems to be more noticeable in weight bearing activities such as running versus a non- weight bearing exercise like cycling or swimming. All of the women I spoke with noticed this, especially in the last trimester of their pregnancies.

The cardiovascular changes in pregnancy are not only influenced by the duration, intensity, and type of exercise you are performing, but also by the position of your body. For instance, some women, when supine (lying on their backs), will develop a drop in blood pressure, causing dizziness and lightheadedness. This happens because while you are on your back, your enlarged uterus puts pressure on the vena cava, a main vein through which blood flows from your body back to your heart. This compression can cause a decrease in blood flow to the uterus. It is recommended that this position be avoided after your fourth month. Prolonged standing without moving can cause similar problems due to a pooling of blood in your legs.

One of the most obvious changes in pregnancy is a steady shift in your center of gravity. Fortunately these changes occur gradually over time and we are "adapting" daily. Nevertheless, it is best to avoid activities where loss of balance may be dangerous, like downhill skiing, speed skating, skateblading, or rock climbing.

Less obvious is the fact that pregnancy hormones relax your joints and ligaments. (Mittelmark, Wiswell, Drinkwater, 1991, p.123) This looseness of ligaments makes you more vulnerable to strains or sprains during exercise. This is especially true for weight bearing activities such as running or aerobics. Lower back pain, which is common in pregnancy, is partly due to a relaxation of your lower back ligaments. (Mittelmark et al. 1991, p. 123)

You can compensate for these changes by modifying your exercise patterns by avoiding such exercises as double-leg raises and straight-leg toe touches that increase the bend in your back. (Prior to pregnancy, you will want to aim for overall body strength and conditioning. Concentrate on your abdominal and back muscles. Practice good posture and proper lifting and bending techniques. The payoff will be a more comfortable pregnancy with less risk of injury.)

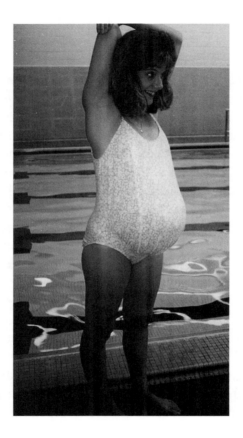

You "adapt" daily to the steady shift in your center of gravity.

Because of all the chemical changes taking place to meet the demands of pregnancy, your basal metabolic rate will normally be higher than before you were pregnant. This will cause you to feel warmer. Then, when you exercise, you will feel even warmer. So how does your body get rid of this heat when you exercise during pregnancy? You sweat. Your increased blood volume helps to cool you and the fetus by transporting warmed blood towards your skin's surface where it is cooled. Sweating makes you feel cooler as water evaporates on your skin's surface. Since your body surface increases in pregnancy (added weight), this cooling response is enhanced even more.

Women who are physically fit seem better able to stay cooler during exercise. (Clapp, 1991) A fit woman's cardiovascular system does a better job of moving blood to working muscles and to the skin's surface for cooling. Trained athletes sweat sooner and sweat more, thus staying cooler than untrained exercisers. But, regardless of your fitness, this is no license to ignore the risk of overheating, especially during early pregnancy.

What is the chance of overheating during exercise and how might this effect the fetus? Vigorous exercise for long periods of time, can raise your core body temperature, which in turn causes the temperature of the fetus to rise. The critical temperature is in excess of 100.4 degrees F (38 degrees C). Some animal studies have seen an association of neural (spinal) tube defects with high body temperature in early pregnancy. (Edwards 1986) Data concerning temperature effects on human fetal development are not clear. Since the fetus can not cool off through perspiration or respiration, be cautious. Limit your outdoor activity in very hot or humid conditions or head for the pool or an air-conditioned health club. Drink plenty of water to avoid dehydration. Avoid hot tubs, saunas and whirlpools, especially in early pregnancy. Don't exercise if you have an illness with a fever. Play it safe.

The growing needs of pregnancy require energy and, roughly translated, that means you need an extra 300 calories a day. When you exercise, you need to eat enough to meet the basic metabolic needs of pregnancy plus the energy requirements of your physical activity. In general, you should eat to appetite and eat a well-balanced diet. Adequate weight gain (See Chapter 4) is a good gauge or indicator that you are keeping up with your caloric needs. Complex carbohydrates are an excellent source of energy and best replace the nutrients lost during exercise (See Chapter 4).

WHAT ABOUT THE FETUS?

Prior to pregnancy, your exercise goals and mood dictated your physical activity. Now that you are pregnant, you need to consider the passenger on board. The health and well being of the fetus is the focus of numerous studies in pregnancy. Let's see how your exercise affects the fetus.

Blood flow and oxygen supply

During exercise, there is a shift of blood flow from your internal organs (including the uterus) to your working muscles (arms, legs). Conflicting results in studies examining blood flow to the uterus prohibit us from drawing any definite conclusions. We do know that the diversion of blood flow from the uterus is probably lessened due to some of the physiological changes in a normal, healthy pregnancy. Your expanded blood volume, increased cardiac output (your heart pumps more per heart beat), and relaxation of your blood vessels helps to compensate and maintain blood flow to the uterus during moderate levels of exercise. So for safety's sake, exercise at moderate levels — leave the vigorous, prolonged workouts until after pregnancy.

The fetal heart rate is a widely used method for studying the well-being of the fetus. Some confusion surrounds the interpretation of the fetal heart rate response to different types of exercise in a healthy pregnancy. During maternal exercise, we see a small rise in the fetal heart rate of 5 to 25 beats per minute. (Artal et al. 1986; Clapp 1985,1993; Dressendorfer et al. 1980) This response may be due to the adaptation of the fetus to the decreased availability of oxygen. Thus far, we think this may be the fetus's physiological response and not associated with adverse effects on the fetus. Another area where there are conflicting opinions is the slowing of the fetal heart rate shortly following maternal exercise. The results of two studies (Carpenter et al. 1988; Webb et al. 1989) offer some clarification to this phenomenon. The incidence of lowered fetal heart rate (bradycardia) is less than 5% and seems to occur during the first two to three minutes following moderate exercise. This decrease may be a response to lowered cardiac output (amount of blood pumped per beat) following a workout. Investigators (Carpenter et al. 1988; Webb et al. 1989) conclude that these responses are usually transient and are more likely to occur following vigorous, intense exercise. Until further studies can clarify this phenomenon, you should avoid prolonged and intense workouts. (See Workout Intensity Level)

Birth weight

Studies comparing babies' birth weights in active and inactive women have been contradictory. Some studies have suggested that women who exercise at high intensities throughout pregnancy have smaller babies. (Naeye 1982; Tafar, Naeye, and Gobezie 1980; Clapp and Capeless 1990) Clapp compared 87 recreational athletes who continued exercise throughout pregnancy to 44 recreational athletes who discontinued exercise before the end of the first trimester. Birth weight for the exercisers was about 300 grams lower, however, the babies were not stunted in their growth — they had less body fat. Other contradictory studies have reported a higher birth weight for mothers who exercised throughout pregnancy. (Hatch et al. 1993) In this study, low-moderate exercisers had babies that weighed about 100 grams more than non-exercisers. At best, we can conclude that exercise type (i.e., weight-bearing versus non-weight-bearing) and intensity may account for some of the discrepancy. In general, adequate maternal weight gain and appropriate fetal growth, are good indicators that your exercise program falls into the "safe" category for the fetus.

Many active women want to know if exercise will cause a miscarriage, premature labor or developmental problems with the fetus. There is no evidence to suggest that moderate exercise in a healthy pregnancy will cause a miscarriage, alter development of the fetus or put you at higher risk for premature labor. (Wolfe et al. 1994) In fact, moderate activity in healthy, well-nourished, pregnant women can actually prevent some health problems like excessive weight gain, poor posture and lower back pain, fatigue and poor body image. Exercise is currently being considered as part of the treatment for pregnant women who develop gestational diabetes, a resistance to insulin's action on glucose uptake during pregnancy. More research using large scale prospective studies is needed to better understand the effects of different exercises during pregnancy and the outcomes during labor and delivery as well as the effects of exercise during postpartum and lactation.

SPORTS AND ACTIVITIES TO AVOID

Avoid any sport or activity which might cause trauma or serious injury to the abdomen. Even if you suffer only a mild injury to your abdomen, this could potentially have more serious consequences for the fetus such as abruption of the placenta (separation of the placenta from the wall of the uterus). Sports to avoid include hockey, football, basketball, soccer, hang gliding, boxing, fencing, water-skiing, and scuba diving. Similarly, because of the risk of falling, stay away from downhill skiing, skateblading, rock climbing, and ice skating in the later months of pregnancy. (Being pregnant can make it difficult to treat injuries due to the potential risks to the fetus from drugs or anesthesia.) Scuba and deep sea diving can expose you to potentially dangerous pressure changes. In case of doubt, use your common sense.

What precautions should you take at high altitudes? The lack of oxygen at higher altitude can put additional stress on you and your fetus. Avoid altitudes over 10,000 feet during pregnancy. Don't hike or ski at elevations above 8,000 feet. Allow yourself 3 to 4 days to acclimate to the altitude prior to exercising.

Flying during pregnancy is safe but most domestic airlines will not permit flying a week before your due date in case you go into labor naturally.

WORKOUT INTENSITY LEVEL

As I have noted, most research agrees that you should avoid vigorous, intense levels of exercise during pregnancy. So how can you determine just what is your level of intensity? Target heart rate has been a popular method to calculate your exercise intensity. To do this you first calculate your resting heart rate. Count your pulse rate first thing in the morning for 10 seconds and then multiply it by 6. Let's say your resting heart rate is 60 and you are a thirty year old woman.

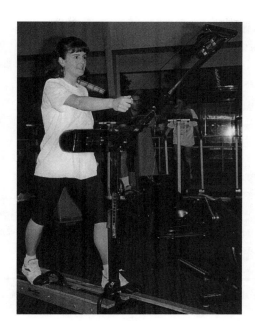

Use the "Talk Test" to monitor your workouts during pregnancy.

Maximal heart rate is the maximum number of beats your heart can beat in one minute. The theoretical figure used is 220 beats per minute. Let's assume you want to exercise at about 70% intensity. (In pregnancy, exercise between 60 to 80% intensity.) Calculate your target heart rate by using the following formula:

        220 (Maximal Heart Rate)
        -30 (Age)
        = 190
        -60 (Resting Heart Rate)
        = 130
        x .70 (Intensity)
        = 91
        +60 (Resting Heart Rate)
        = 151 TARGET HEART RATE

Unfortunately, the target heart rate calculation has some draw-backs in pregnancy. Resting heart rate in pregnancy is normally higher and it is unclear what maximal heart rate is for pregnancy. A better measure of exercise intensity might be Rating of Perceived Exertion (RPE) as developed by Borg, a Swedish physiologist. Using this method, you can correlate your perceived activity level with exertion and aerobic activity. The scale goes from 6 to 20; 6 - 7 being very, very light workouts and 19 - 20 being very, very, hard. Be as accurate as you can when estimating your feelings of exertion. During pregnancy, you should stay around 12-14, (somewhat hard) when exercising. At this intensity of exercise, you should be able to pass the "Talk Test" and easily carry on a conversation while exercising.

RATING OF PERCEIVED EXERTION SCALE

How does the exercise feel?	Rating
	6
Very, very light	7
	8
Very light	9
	10
Fairly light	11
	12
Somewhat Hard	13
	14
Hard	15
	16
Very hard	17
	18
Very, very hard	19
	20

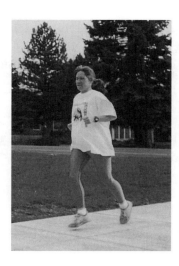

You need to slow down and listen to your body.

WARNING SIGNS

After establishing your exercise program with the guidance of your health provider, you need to recognize warning signs that may alert you to a problem. The following signs and symptoms tell you to stop exercising and to consult your provider.

Pain
Unfortunately, many well-conditioned athletes are used to discomfort during workouts. You need to slow down and listen to your body as it moves from discomfort to pain. "No pain, no gain" does not apply during pregnancy.

Bleeding
Any vaginal bleeding or spotting at any time in pregnancy means STOP and contact your health care provider immediately.

<u>Dizziness, Shortness of Breath, Palpitations, Faint-</u>
<u>ness, or Rapid Heartbeat</u>
Any one of these symptoms is a signal to stop exercising.

<u>Pubic Pain</u>
This may signal irritation, or if persistent, a more serious injury to the pubic bone due to loosening of ligaments.

<u>Rupture of Uterine Membranes (Leaking</u>
<u>Amniotic Fluid) or Regular Uterine Contractions</u>
Stop exercising. Call your health care provider.

While most women can continue to exercise during their pregnancy, there are those who have to cease activity altogether. Here is a runner's story about how she went from an active person to one who had to lie in bed, weeks at a time, during her last two pregnancies.

Exercise is an integral piece of my life. I began running in high school and until I had my children, I was running five times a week, usually four miles or less. I frequently mixed my running with some sort of aerobics and spot exercises. My exercise has always been for my own fulfillment and happiness — I rarely compete in races and therefore do not think of it as training for an event. Instead, it is a necessity of my life.

I ran during the initial half of my first pregnancy and then, because of discomfort, I switched to swimming. I swam at least five times a week up until the week that my daughter was born.

When I began my second pregnancy, I was attending aerobics classes and walking three to four miles a day with a stroller. I was in great shape and did not expect to have any difficulties. But at seventeen weeks, I suddenly developed complications.

I was diagnosed as having placenta previa (the placenta was covering my cervix), and after a few days in the hospital, was sent home to rest. Things got worse and within a week I developed placental abruption (the placenta was coming off the uterine wall and causing fairly heavy bleeding). I entered the hospital and was on my side in bed for ten weeks.

Being immobile and unable to get outside drove me crazy, but I was so concerned with saving the pregnancy and the baby that I did not dwell on the subject. I approached it as a contest — the longer I could lie still, the closer I came to the prize. But there was no assurance of a happy ending. I was facing a possible life-threatening hemorrhage as well as a premature child. My pregnancy ended at twenty-eight weeks and my son died within hours of his birth. As painful as this was, I would have been in more pain had he lived with an extreme disability.

In three months, I had regained my strength and was running and taking aerobics classes on a regular schedule. I was possessed to shed the extra pounds and erase my inactivity to lessen the pain of what I had been through. By three months postpartum, I had regained most of my fitness although I felt more drained than revitalized by exercise. In hindsight, giving myself extra time might have been healthier.

I was determined to get on with having a sibling for my daughter and was buoyed by the doctor's promise that there was a 95% chance that the next pregnancy would be healthy and normal. I did not delay — I was pregnant four and a half months from leaving the hospital.

I delayed my initial visit to the obstetrician because I was afraid that the doctor would restrict my activity. At eight weeks, I made the visit and was restricted to walking. By thirteen weeks, I was repeating the events of my second pregnancy and was on limited activity, when then progressed to bed rest by about twenty weeks.

This was such a horrible series of events that I functioned in a fog for weeks. My husband and doctors and I had long talks — there were no promises and we all knew it. I was further along in the pregnancy and the symptoms were less severe so I was hopeful and wanted to continue. After premature labor and a ten-day hospital stay, I went home with a portable monitor for contractions and instructions to stay in bed.

It took every ounce of self-control and mental strength which I could gather to stay in bed this time around, even though I was at home. I found that you basically just have to tough it out and look forward to getting up again. Fortunately, it was worth it — our little boy was born early, but healthy, after thirty-four weeks.

Walking was my first activity after bed rest. Pushing a double stroller holding thirty-eight pounds of children made a decent workout. One of the largest issues for me was that since my son was six weeks premature, he was on a heart and respiration monitor. I did not want to leave him with anyone other than my husband for quite a few months after his birth.

After several months, I was ready to start running again. Rather than wait for my husband to come home, which would mean running late and in the dark, I packed up the children and toys and drove in mid-day to a lightly used track. I placed my son's car seat in the middle of the inner track — where I could see him and hear his monitor if it went off — and set my daughter up with toys on a blanket near him. I then ran laps around them. A good day would be being able to complete three miles with only one stop per mile. A more typical routine was an interruption every lap or two. Mentally, it drove me crazy. Physically, it was good for me.

I am used to juggling my day a bit to accommodate exercise but now, with two children, it was harder to do so. My husband's travel and work schedule make it tough for him to help during the week and I was having trouble lining up baby-sitters. Therefore, I chose to exercise at places which provide sitting. I took aerobics classes as my primary form of exercise until my son turned four. I still ran when I had the chance, but aerobics helped keep me in excellent shape.

Now, I can fit my running in while my son is at preschool. I still have to adjust to large gaps in my workout schedule. There's not much you can do when the children get the flu and chicken pox, back to back. Life is just different now than before children.

The best part of my bed rest is my son and the added appreciation it gives me for the lives of both our children.

Here is the story of a thirty-two year old runner who also had to stop exercising during her first pregnancy.

Here's my story. After a weekend of fatigue (more than usual) and an incidence of seeing "floaters," my husband took my blood pressure and found it elevated. When I called the O.B. office with my reading, they said that they wanted me to come in right away. When I got to the office, my blood pressure was even more elevated and I they diagnosed pregnancy-induced hypertension — and wanted to hospitalize me right away. I was devastated.

Until this point (32 weeks), I'd had such a healthy and active pregnancy. My physician even said that she wanted to make me a "poster child" for pregnancy with the slogan, "Yes, there is life during pregnancy." I felt like I had been doing all the right things to keep myself mentally and physically fit. I just could not believe that this was happening! I kept thinking that I must have done something wrong.

For the first time during my pregnancy, I felt as if every-thing was out of my control. The physician and nurses assured me that this was not my fault, that the cause of pregnancy-induced hypertension was unknown, and that 5-10% of women get it during their first pregnancy. They gave me some literature that explained the condition in more detail. I also searched through my own "volumes" of prenatal material to learn all that I could about this condition. The information that I found was similar to that which the doctor gave me but I think that doing some re-search on my own helped me feel a little more in control of the situation. And, since I was on "bedrest," I had plenty of time to read. To pass the time and help myself gain a better sense of control, I laid there and made plans for my post-partum exercise program.

I got a lot of help and understanding from my husband during this period. He did everything at home that needed to be done to insure that I got complete bed rest. He brought books and playing cards to the hospital and tracked down several excellent prenatal videos. (We had been able to attend only one of our prenatal classes before my hyper-tension hit.)

After our son was born, I followed my physician's advice and eased back into exercise. I didn't want to push things too much after the bout with elevated blood pressure but I did get out and start walking during the first week after giving birth, with the baby in a front carrier. The fresh air and movement were good for our son and me.

After four weeks, I was ready for some more vigorous ex-ercise. My husband and I had to get a little creative about scheduling exercise times and took turns going out, some-times very early in the morning. Exercise is something very important (physically and mentally) for both of us so we made it a priority.

We also got creative about how we exercised. We bought a running stroller and my husband took our son out in it for not only a workout, but to give me a break and allow me some time to exercise. I "wore" my son in the front carrier at the gym while I used the stair machine. It gave an added benefit to my workout while it lulled the baby to sleep. Now that our son is older, we have a back carrier and hike and cross-country ski with him in tow.

Exercising is certainly not the same since our son was born. However, with some careful planning and teamwork, there is exercise A.B. (After Baby) I dare say that perhaps the exercise is more rewarding because of the extra effort that goes into the planning.

** "Sidelines" — a non-profit network provides support and information for bedridden women. (714) 497-2265.

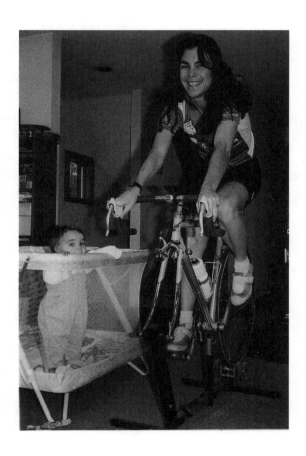

Exercise A.B. (After Baby) takes some extra planning.

SETTING YOUR OWN GUIDELINES

As you read this book, you'll hear from women who continued to run, cycle, canoe, or ski throughout their pregnancies. You'll hear from others who had to slow down, change activities, or even stop exercising altogether. Just as each of us is different, each of our pregnancies will be different. That's why you must individualize your exercise program and set it up under the guidance of your health provider. Here are some exercise tips to consider when you do:

1. Listen to your body. Now is the time to tune in to all the signals and cues.
2. Be prepared to adapt and modify your program. Be flexible!
3. Rest. Any exercise program should be balanced by adequate rest.
4. Eat! Maintain a balanced diet with adequate calories. Let your appetite guide you.
5. Avoid high intensity workouts. Slow and easy ... keep it 12-14 on the RPE scale.
6. Avoid overheating and drink plenty of fluids.
7. Recognize warning signs tostop exercising.

4

NUTRITION

Your pregnancy will be a period in your life when you will be showered with attention. You'll get congratulatory greetings, inquiries about your health, comments on how big or small you are, and keen observations on every morsel you put in your mouth. Discerning eyes will never fail to capture you when you are surrendering to that dish of ice cream or an extra slice of pizza. But it's up to you to "eat for two" wisely.

What you eat or don't eat during pregnancy is important: it affects your health and the growing needs of your developing baby. For example, a diet deficient in essential nutrients may result in a low birth weight baby who is at risk for delivery complications, infection, or impaired intelligence. Conversely, a well-balanced diet, both before and during pregnancy, increases your chances of delivering a healthy normal weight baby. No one's diet is perfect, but certainly during your pregnancy you should plan your diet carefully and focus on "quality."

Are you concerned about weight gain? It's not unusual — many physically active and athletic women exercise to control their weight. Competitive athletes are keenly aware of weight gain and may restrict themselves calorically by following a very low fat diet. Because of this, these women may also be deficient in certain vitamins and minerals, especially iron.

Ideally, the time for you to establish a healthy pattern of eating is <u>before</u> pregnancy. There is evidence that a diet deficient in folic acid may contribute to neural tube defects (spina bifida). Current guidelines recommend that childbearing women should consume 0.4 mg of folic acid a day. You can meet this by eating a diet rich in leafy vegetables, whole grains, eggs, oranges and legumes.

EATING FOR TWO

Most of you have probably eagerly planned for your pregnancy. At the same time, if you are physically active, you have concerns about how your pregnancy will affect your body. In particular, you are probably worried about weight gain and how you will lose the weight afterwards. Of the women I see in my practice, one of their biggest fears is getting "fat" and then not losing the weight because of lack of exercise due to the demands of parenting.

The apprehension of becoming fat probably exists for most of us during our lifetime, sometimes starting with adolescence and continuing into adulthood. During pregnancy, this concern can be magnified. I know that during my pregnancy I didn't want to gain excessive weight because I wanted to stay fit both during and after the pregnancy. On the other hand, my goal was to gain "nutritiously" and grow a healthy baby.

WHAT IS A HEALTHY WEIGHT GAIN?

For the average woman, weight gain is usually between 25 and 35 pounds. If you are underweight, you may gain more toward the high end, and if you are overweight, more toward the lower end. The pattern of gain is also important. A three to four pound gain during the first trimester, followed by a twelve to fourteen pound gain in the second trimester is reasonable. After this, a pound a week during the last three months will put you at your goal.

ESTIMATED BREAKDOWN OF WEIGHT GAIN DURING PREGNANCY

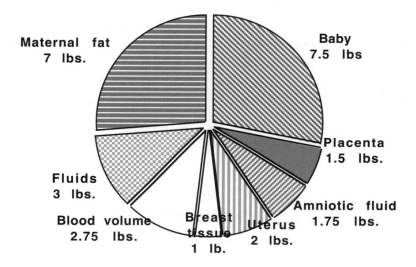

Maternal fat
7 lbs.

Baby
7.5 lbs

Placenta
1.5 lbs.

Fluids
3 lbs.

Amniotic fluid
1.75 lbs.

Blood volume
2.75 lbs.

Breast
tissue
1 lb.

Uterus
2 lbs.

QUALITY COUNTS

Eating a healthy diet during your pregnancy will reap many rewards for you and your baby. A balanced diet will help improve your mood swings and boost your energy level while it improves the odds of delivering a healthy baby.

This "healthy eating" responsibility may feel overwhelming at times, especially if you had an unbalanced diet before pregnancy. Why not think of pregnancy as training for an athletic event — the birth of your baby? Make a proper diet an integral part of your training.

EXPECTANT EATING

In pregnancy, we require an additional 300 calories a day, for the growing fetus and for the energy needs of just being pregnant. When you think about it, 300 calories does not really add up to a feeding frenzy. A bran muffin and a cup of yogurt adds up to this "extra." The challenge is to create a balanced energizing diet. The first step is to look at your current diet. Keep track of everything you eat or drink for several days (be honest!) and see how your daily intake stacks up to the Food Guide Pyramid. I think the food pyramid is easy to follow and creates a visual picture of how you should structure your daily menus.

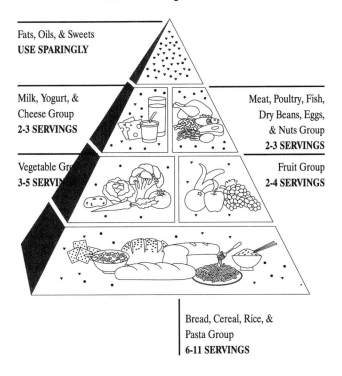

Food Guide Pyramid
A Guide to Daily Food Choices

Fats, Oils, & Sweets
USE SPARINGLY

Milk, Yogurt, &
Cheese Group
2-3 SERVINGS

Meat, Poultry, Fish,
Dry Beans, Eggs,
& Nuts Group
2-3 SERVINGS

Vegetable Gr
3-5 SERVI

Fruit Group
2-4 SERVINGS

Bread, Cereal, Rice, &
Pasta Group
6-11 SERVINGS

Source: U.S. Department of Agriculture/U.S. Department of Health and Human Services

BREAD GROUP - A serving is equal to one slice of bread, 1/2 cup rice, 1/2 cup pasta. Concentrate on whole grains.
VEGETABLE GROUP- A serving is equal to 1/2 cup of cooked vegetable, 1 cup of leafy raw vegetable. Concentrate on leafy green and deep yellow vegetables.
FRUIT GROUP- A serving is equal to one medium apple or 1/2 grapefruit
MILK GROUP- A serving is equal to 1 cup of milk, 1 cup of yogurt or 2 oz. of cheese
MEAT GROUP- A serving is equal to 2 to 3 oz. of lean meat, fish or poultry. Choose lean cuts, avoid frying.

DIET FOR THE ACTIVE PREGNANCY

There has been little research on the nutritional needs of physically active women in pregnancy. The energy needs of active pregnant women varies with the type of activity you are performing, its duration, and your stage in the pregnancy. It is impossible to provide specific guidelines due to all of these variables. Basically, if you "eat to appetite" (eat when you are hungry, stop when you are full), you will fulfill the energy needs of your physical activity and growing needs of your baby. You should concentrate on complex carbohydrates (whole grain breads, cereals, rice, vegetables, dried beans and peas). Your weight gain will help you determine if you are taking in enough calories. If you begin to lose weight, or fail to gain, this is an indicator that you need to examine closely your diet and make the necessary changes to gain adequate weight. Reviewing a two or three day diet recall is an easy way to do this. If you are lactose intolerant or do not drink milk, you may need to take a calcium supplement. A discussion with your health provider about your exercise program and diet is important. You want to be sure that both you and your baby are gaining and "growing nutritiously."

AFTER THE BABY

One of the first concerns of most women after delivery is getting back to their prepregnancy weight. Remember, it took you nine months to gain the weight so it will take a bit of time to lose it. A common mistake some women make is to starve themselves to achieve a rapid weight loss. This approach has a price to pay.

In the weeks following delivery, your body is undergoing some significant changes. The uterus is shrinking, your blood volume is decreasing, and hormones are dropping to their nonpregnant levels (unless you are nursing). All of this change, plus the arrival of your new baby who depends on you and your partner for everything, can feel overwhelming. Some women experience "postpartum blues." These "down" feelings can occur as early as the third day postpartum or any time during the first year. One of the major causes is probably due to the tremendous shift in hormones and fatigue. Interrupted sleep is one of the biggest challenges new parents have to cope with. We'll talk more about this later, but a healthy diet will help you survive these first few months.

If you are breastfeeding, you need an additional 400-500 calories a day (Cunningham et al. 1993, p.256). This extra energy will assure an adequate milk supply. Breastfeeding demands the same scrutiny of your diet you had during pregnancy. You can excrete substances from what you eat or drink in your breast milk. Limiting your caffeine or alcohol intake is wise. Be sure to question the safety of over the counter or prescription drugs with your health provider. If you were taking a prenatal vitamin supplement, you can continue taking this while nursing.

Be sure to talk to your health care provider about both your exercise program and your diet. It's not always easy to be objective about your own eating habits, especially when that hot fudge sundae is screaming your name, so it's good to get an outside opinion. Your nutrition game plan is an important part of a fit pregnancy and after.

5

STRETCHING

As a fit woman, you are well aware of the importance of proper warm-up, stretching and cool down routines in your exercise program. Unfortunately, this awareness does not always get translated into practice. I know the excuses because I've used most of them: "I'm in a hurry; I'll stretch later; This feels too easy; I'd rather be working out." Now, during pregancy, it's more important than ever to include a few simple routines into pregnancy and post-pregnancy fitness programs. Why risk injury by launching too quickly into a workout? Warming up and cooling down routines are a good investment of your time.

WARMUP/COOLDOWN ROUTINES

In Chapter 2, we first mentioned that pregnancy hormones make your joints and ligaments more relaxed and vulnerable to injury. When you warm up, you raise the temperature of your muscles, route more blood to your muscles, and increase the synovial fluid (a fluid that lubricates) in your joints (Anderson, B. 1980). You prepare your tendons, ligaments, and muscles for the work ahead.

A warm-up can be as simple as jogging 5 to 10 minutes prior

to running, doing a few easy laps in the pool, or spinning your wheels on the bike for a few miles. The idea is to slowly get specific muscles warmed up and ready for the workout.

Is stretching the same as warming up? No, it is not. After a brief warm-up, you can gently stretch the major muscles that you will be using in your workout. For instance, in running you would focus on your calf, quadriceps, and hamstring muscles before the run, saving the bulk of your stretching for after your workout when your muscles will be warmed and more flexible.

Cooling down, or slowing down, is the best way to end your workout. Cooling down slowly lowers your heart rate and reduces muscle soreness. A slow jog around the corner, a few easy laps of breast stroke, or walking in place after aerobics is all it takes to lead into your post-exercise stretching routine. Towel off or change into dry clothes beforehand if necessary. Grab something to drink and start your stretching routine.

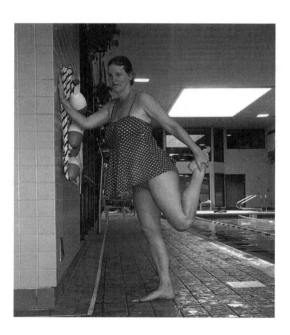

Stretching relaxes your muscles, promotes better circulation, and helps you stay flexible.

PROPER STRETCHING

Like warm-ups and cool-downs, stretching is easy to skip over when you are short on time. However, now, more than ever, you should pledge to take the time to stretch. Stretching has a lot of positive benefits: it relaxes your muscles, promotes better circulation, and helps you stay flexible. It also keeps you focused on your changing body as you take the time to stretch specific muscle groups. Stretching relaxes your muscles and your mind.

Stretching is easy, but learn to do it properly. Improper stretching can cause injury to joints, ligaments or muscles during and after your pregnancy. Bob Anderson, in his book, *Stretching*, offers the following tips. Never force a stretch to the point of pain. Avoid bouncing. Instead, try for a relaxed, slow stretch. Breathe in and out slowly and don't hold your breath. Begin a stretch by holding it for 10 to 30 seconds, then stretch a little further. You should feel some mild tension but not pain. Hold the stretch for another 10 to 30 seconds. Listen to your body along the way and make adjustments as necessary.

PREGNANCY STRETCHES

There are some excellent books on stretching. A particularly good one is *Stretching* by Bob Anderson (See Reference List). Most likely you have your own stretching routine already in place that you can modify both during and after your pregnancy. The following are stretches that are especially good during pregnancy.

Neck Rolls
- Can be done sitting or standing
- Drop your head to the right, slowly roll your head forward and then to your left shoulder.
- Repeat several times.

Shoulder Rolls
- Can be done sitting or standing.
- Move your right shoulder forward, up and then down and back, making a full circle. Repeat with your left shoulder.
- Do 5 reps each side.

Arm Reaches
- Stand or sit.
- Inhale as you raise your right arm above your head, stretching from the waist. Exhale as you bring your arm down.
- Repeat on the left side.
- Do 5 reps on each side.

Arm Stretches
- Can be done standing or sitting.
- Raise your right arm over your head, bending it at the elbow, and place your hand on your back.
- Grab your elbow with your left hand and gently pull back. You should feel the stretch along your upper arm.
- Hold the stretch for 10 to 30 seconds, then stretch a little further for another 10 to 30 seconds.
- Repeat on your left arm.
- For the outer arm muscles, bring your right arm straight across your chest.
- Place your left hand on your elbow and gently pull your arm closer to your chest.
- Hold for 10 to 30 seconds and then stretch a little further for another 10 to 30 seconds.
- Repeat on your left arm.

Chest Stretch
- Stand with your feet slightly apart.
- Lace your fingers together behind your back.
- Slowly lift your hands up behind you, pulling your shoulder blades together and keeping your head level.
- Hold for 10 to 30 seconds and then stretch a little further or another 10 to 30 seconds.

Kegel Exercise
- Helps to strengthen muscles that support your bladder, uterus, and rectum.
- Can be done lying down, sitting, or standing.
- Tighten and release the muscles around your vagina. (Try this exercise while urinating by starting and then stopping the flow of urine.)
- Work up to 25 contractions.

Super Kegels
- Instead of tightening and then releasing your pelvic muscles, try holding these muscles as tight as possible for 10 to 20 seconds. This is more effective if done one at a time.
- Try the exercise 10 times over the course of a day.

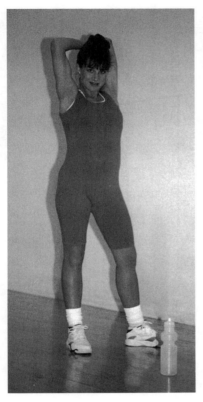

Arm Stretch

Pelvic Tilt
- Helps relieve back ache and can be done standing or kneeling on all fours
- Stand comfortably.
- Inhale and relax. Exhale and pull your buttocks under and forward. Hold for the count of 5. You can also do this pressing the small of your back against a wall.
- Do 5 reps.

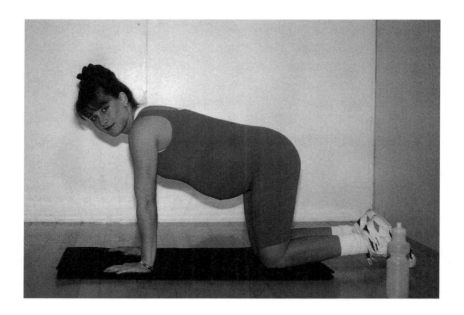

Pelvic Tilt

Pelvic Tilt -kneeling
- Kneel on your hands and knees.
- Keep a flat back. Inhale and relax. Exhale and pull your buttocks under and forward while feeling your abdomen tightening. Hold for the count of 5.
- Do 5 reps.

Butterfly/Groin Stretch
- Sit on the floor with the soles of your feet together.
- Hold your ankles. Bring your feet as close to your body as comfortable while keeping your back straight.
- Inhale and relax. Exhale and lower yourself forward.
- Hold the stretch easy for 10 to 30 seconds, then stretch a little further for another 10 to 30 seconds.
- Squatting is a good stretch for your inner thigh and calf muscles.
- Squat down, keeping your back straight.
- Try to keep your heels on the floor while you balance yourself evenly on flat feet.

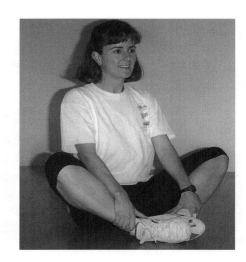

Butterfly/Groin Stretch

Leg Stretches
- Sit on the floor with your left leg stretched out to the side, your foot flexed, and your other leg drawn in.
- Face forward and lean your body toward the outstretched leg.
- Lift your right arm over your head and with your left hand grasp your ankle or calf.
- Hold the stretch for 10 to 30 seconds, then stretch a little further for another 10 to 30 seconds.
- Repeat on the right side.

Side Leg Stretches
- Lie on your right side with your legs straight or with the lower leg bent at the knee.
- Support your head with your right hand and place your left hand in front of you. Inhale and relax.
- Keep your foot flexed as you raise your left leg as high as you can,then exhale as you slowly lower it.
- Repeat ten times then roll to your left side and repeat ten times.
- You can also do this with your top leg bent at the knee so your leg is at a right angle to your body. Remember to keep your foot flexed as you raise and lower your leg.

Calf Stretches
- Stand facing a wall.
- Bend one knee and bring it toward the wall.
- Keep your back leg straight with your foot facing forward.
- Press your heel to the floor.
- Feel the stretch in your calf muscle.
- Hold for 10 to 30 seconds then stretch a little further for another
  10 to 30 seconds. Stretch the other calf.
  Another easy way to stretch your calf muscle is on a stair step.
- Stand on the edge of a step with your legs straight and your
  heels hanging over the edge.
- Transfer your weight to one leg and lower that heel. For balance,
  hold on to a wall or rail.
- Hold the stretch for 10 to 30 seconds. Repeat on the other leg.
- To specifically stretch your soleus muscle in your calf, do this
  stretch with a bent knee as you lower your heel.

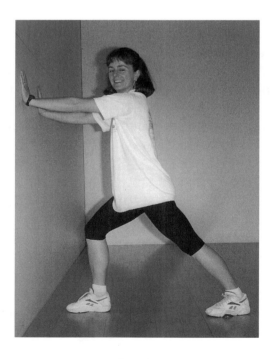

Calf Stretch

Lunge Stretch
- Bring your right leg forward and bend your knee, keeping your foot facing straight.
- Your leg should be at a right angle to the floor.
- Support your body with your hands on the floor.
- Stretch your left leg behind you while pushing your hips down toward the floor.
- Hold this stretch for 10 to 30 seconds.
- Switch legs and repeat.

Hamstrings
- From a standing position, place your right foot in front of you.
- Push down your heel as you pull your toes up toward you.
- Try to keep your leg straight and back flat. Bend your left leg for support.
- Feel the stretch along the back of your leg.
- Hold for 10 to 30 seconds, then stretch a little further to 10 to 30 seconds.
- Repeat with your right leg.

Quadriceps Stretch
- Stand next to a wall or chair for support.
- Bend your left knee and with your right hand, pull your heel straight back toward your buttocks.
- Keep your thigh parallel to your other leg.
- Hold for 10 to 30 seconds and then stretch a little further for another 10 to 30 seconds.
- Repeat on your right leg.

Stretching is one way to help you stay flexible and relaxed. Yoga and massage are other options. Yoga classes designed for pregnancy are very beneficial. The gentle stretching and focused breathing patterns in yoga are ideal for pregnancy and childbirth preparation. See if there are any prenatal yoga classes in your area.

Massage is a comforting technique which relieves muscle tension, improves flexibility and increases circulation. Many athletes include sport massage in their training as a way to promote recovery and reduce the risk of injury. Massage therapy helps remove lactic acid, a byproduct of anaerobic exercise, which is believed to cause muscle soreness. When done correctly, massage provides a feeling of relaxation and well-being. A massage by your partner or friend offers relief to tense shoulders, lower back ache and other pregnancy trouble spots. Massage should be avoided if you have a history of phlebitis or blood clots.

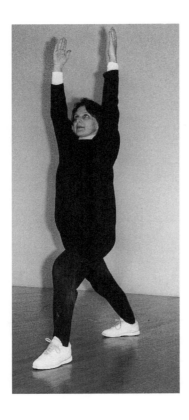

The gentle stretching and focused breathing patterns in yoga are ideal for pregnancy and childbirth preparation.

Stretching feels good. Proper stretching relaxes your muscles, reduces tension, promotes circulation, keeps you flexible and prevents injury. Tailor your stretching routine to your own body signals and tight spots; runners might focus more on their legs and hips while swimmers and paddlers stretch more of their upper bodies. No two bodies are the same and pregnancy will likely cause new "trouble spots," such as your back, hips and pelvis. Stretching will offer relief and help you relax mentally and physically. It's time well spent.

6

AEROBICS

The research and writing of Dr. Kenneth Cooper helped to create the aerobic exercise movement in this country. Aerobic means "using oxygen" which happens every time we perform an exercise like running, walking, cycling, or aerobic dance. Our body meets the challenge of sustaining physical activity by improving its ability to get oxygen from our lungs to our working muscles. This is what we call cardiovascular fitness. Dr. Cooper's belief in the physical and emotional benefits of aerobic exercise started Americans moving aerobically.

Aerobic dance first gained popularity in the seventies. Jackie Sorenson was one of the early designers of choreographed movements to music. As its popularity grew, new forms evolved: Jazzercise™, Dancercise™, low impact, high impact and bench step aerobics. Today, many women like yourself attend aerobics classes on a regular basis at health clubs, aerobics studios, YWCA's and in your own home with videotapes.

Women join aerobics classes for many reasons. "Exercise helps keep me fit and toned and gives me an energy boost," says Karen, a mother of two. She attends an aerobics class three times a week at a local health club. For many women, aerobics is a fun way to get exercise. There's class camaraderie, the diversion of music and an enthusiastic instructor to motivate you and lead you through the workout. By attending a well-designed aerobics class at least three times a week, you will improve your cardiovascular fitness and flexibility, strengthen and tone your muscles and leave your workouts with a relaxed, yet invigorated feeling.

WHAT MAKES A GOOD AEROBICS CLASS?

The instructor

Your instructor should be knowledgeable, enthusiastic, and preferably certified. There are several organizations which offer certification including The Aerobics and Fitness Association of America (AFAA), The American Council on Exercise (ACE), and the American College of Sports Medicine (ACSM). The instructor has the responsibility of conducting a safe class and monitoring the intensity of the workout during the aerobic phase of the class. He or she should teach participants how to calculate their target heart rate. (220 minus your age = Maximum Heart Rate. Maximum Heart Rate x (60% to 75%) = Target Heart Rate.)

The class

All classes, (low impact, high impact and bench step aerobics) generally follow a similar format. Low impact classes are less stressful to your joints by keeping leg and foot motions low to the ground. One foot remains on the floor at all times. High impact includes more jumping and hopping while bench step aerobics incorporates choreographed stepping movements on and off a platform. Each of these classes starts with a warm-up/stretching phase which slowly warms up all of your major muscle groups. Warmed, flexible muscles are less prone to injury. Your pulse rate slowly rises in preparation for the work ahead.

The cardiovascular phase is usually 20 to 60 minutes of choreographed arm and leg movements which raises your heart rate. Periodically checking your pulse lets you know if you are working at your target heart rate. By keeping your exercising heart rate close to your target heart rate, you will be "utilizing oxygen" more

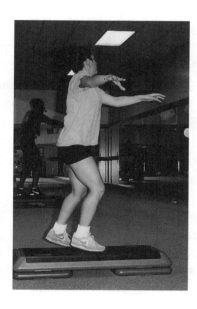

Bench step aerobics incorporates choreographed
stepping movements on and off a platform.

efficiently and becoming more fit. You gradually slow your movements down and lower your pulse rate as you begin the strength and toning phase.

This workout phase targets specific muscle groups to build strength and improve tone for both your upper and lower body. Hand held weights or stretch bands can add resistance to this part of the workout. When using weights or stretch bands, avoid holding your breath. Exhale during the contraction of the muscle and inhale during the release. We'll cover this in more detail in the next chapter.

The cool down phase incorporates slow, rhythmic movements to lower your heart rate and prevent blood from pooling in your extremities. This is followed by stretching all your major muscle groups while breathing slowly and deeply. Kathryn Caiello, a personal fitness trainer and aerobics instructor, emphasizes the importance of the stretching portion of the class. "Stretching helps promote muscle balance and flexibility and prevents muscle soreness. Don't be tempted to skip it."

The facility

Try to find a facility with an aerobics room large enough to accommodate all participants. Look for wooden or tightly carpeted floor surfaces (no concrete) as well as air-conditioning and good ventilation. Make sure that there are drinking water and bathroom facilities nearby. The facility should have mirrors to help check for correct body positions and to increase the visibility of the instructor. Good acoustics and an adequate sound system are also important considerations.

AEROBICS FOR TWO

The primary goal of any prenatal fitness program is the safety of you and your fetus. Before you became pregnant, your exercise goals might have been to stay trim and toned and perhaps to lose weight. Routines you may have used then, the intense, vigorous workouts designed to reduce weight, are not safe now that you are pregnant. Most studies agree that prenatal exercise programs should be low impact and moderate intensity. Let's look at how you can still use aerobics to stay fit.

A well-designed prenatal aerobics class which takes into account your body's tremendous physical changes can offer many benefits during your pregnancy. You can reduce backache, swelling, pelvic pressure, excessive weight gain, and fatigue. You can maintain your aerobic fitness and muscular strength and flexibility. An active, moving body also enhances self-esteem and builds self confidence.

"Exercise really lifts my spirits and helps me feel positive about getting larger," reports Maria a twenty-four year old graduate student expecting her first child. She attends a prenatal aerobics class twice a week.

A prenatal aerobics class should be taught by a certified instructor who is trained in the physiology, anatomy and biomechanics of pregnancy. Classes should be individualized and follow the current 1994 ACOG guidelines for exercise in pregnancy (See Chapter 3). Before starting a class, discuss your plans with your health care provider who is familiar with your fitness level, medical history, and the health of your pregnancy.

Specialized classes for pregnant women provide closer individual monitoring in a supportive environment. You can discuss pregnancy-related topics and experiences shared by the group. "I am at the end of my eighth month and definitely feel stronger and more confident about my pregnancy because of the prenatal aerobics class. I have gained weight in the right places and not the wrong ones," reports Diane, expecting her first child.

GENERAL GUIDELINES FOR PRENATAL AEROBICS

As mentioned previously, you need to discuss your exercise plans with your health care provider. Let your instructor know of any special concerns or recent developments in your pregnancy. Eat a light snack about an hour before class. Drink plenty of fluids and bring your water bottle to class. Remember, you sweat more in pregnancy so dress in light, breathable clothing. Layering is a good idea so you can peel off as you warm up. Avoid exercising in hot, humid conditions or if you have a fever. Wear a panty liner if you have vaginal discharge or problems with leaking urine. A good supportive bra is important. Shoes designed for aerobics are best. Listen to your body. Exercise according to how you feel and not how you think you should be exercising.

Your changing body requires modification of exercises to avoid injury or discomfort. The hormones of pregnancy make your joints and ligaments more relaxed and vulnerable to strain or sprains. Your added weight changes your posture causing you to lean forward slightly. In turn, this shift in your center of gravity causes some muscles in your body to relax and others to tighten. A prenatal aerobics class must modify certain exercises, especially to those areas of your body under "mechanical stress" such as your abdomen, pelvis, back and hips.

ABDOMINAL EXERCISE MODIFICATIONS

You should modify abdominal exercises after the fourth month to avoid putting direct pressure on the abdominal muscles. For example, you can do abdominal curl-ups in a semirecumbent position with knees rolled to the side. Crossing your arms over your abdomen can provide additional support to the abdominal wall.

Also, you should keep in mind that exercising from the supine position (flat on your back) causes the weight of your uterus to compress the vena cava, a large vein that returns blood from your lower body to your heart. This can cause a drop in blood pressure (supine hypotension) making you feel dizzy or faint.

Diastasis recti is the complete or partial separation of the rectus abdominis muscle. Most common in the third trimester of pregnancy, it is caused by weak abdominal muscles, a big baby, obesity, heredity, and other factors. You can measure the degree of separation. Ask your health provider to teach you how to check for this. Avoid abdominal work if there is a separation of these muscles.

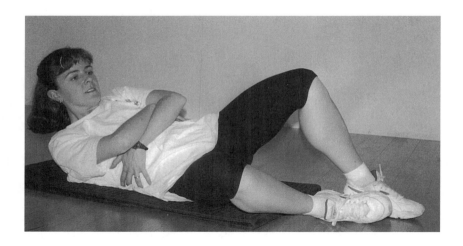

Modify abdominal exercises after the fourth month to avoid putting direct pressure on the abdominal muscles.

PELVIC EXERCISE MODIFICATIONS

The pelvic floor refers to the muscles and fascia that support your pelvic organs, the bladder, uterus, and rectum. During pregnancy, leaking of urine can be a sign of weakness in these muscles. The Kegel exercise is an isometric contraction of these muscles. You can learn this by trying to hold your flow of urine midstream.

Once you are able to effectively isolate these muscles, you can incorporate Kegels into abdominal and buttocks exercises. I remind women to do Kegel exercises at every stoplight while driving. As you'll read later, it is good to continue Kegels after pregnancy.

Large ligaments help support your expanding uterus. The constant stretching of these ligaments can cause irritation, especially with sudden movements. Again, modified abdominal exercises will reduce discomfort. Keep your knee and hip joints slightly bent while doing hip abductions (leg moving outward) and hip adductions (leg moving inward). Instead of using the "all fours" position for buttocks exercises, try standing for working these muscles. Move slowly from side to side and practice proper body mechanics by using your arms when rising from the floor.

BACKACHES

As your pregnancy advances, the weight of your uterus pulls your pelvis forward causing you to curve your lower back, round your shoulders, and lean your head forward. This postural change causes lower backache. Exercises should focus on strengthening your back, hip and abdominal muscles as well as stretching and relaxing the back, shoulders and neck. The cat stretch is an easy back stretch to do. Get on all fours (hands and knees) and round your back toward the ceiling as you exhale. Inhale as you lower your back to a flat position. The cat stretch can also relieve strain to the pelvic ligaments.

MUSCLE CRAMPS

You can trigger muscle cramps in your thighs or calves by pointing your toes during a routine. They are also common at night when you are suddenly awakened by a pain in your calf muscle. Relief will come by stretching the muscle and holding it until the cramp subsides. Straighten your knee for a hamstring cramp and dorsiflex your foot (pull back the toes) for a calf cramp.

PRENATAL CLASS FORMAT

Let's talk about a prenatal class format designed for the "two" of you.

<u>Warm-up</u>

As we mentioned in the previous chapter, gentle stretching and range of motion exercises helps get your joints, ligaments and muscles ready for movement. Focus attention on your vulnerable areas: your pelvic ligaments, your lower back and your hips. Stretch to the point of mild tension, not pain. Breathe in and out slowly. Avoid holding your breath.

Aerobics (non-impact)

Avoid bouncy, jerky movements and sudden changes in direction. Movements should be smooth and controlled. Pay attention to good posture. Keep your legs moving while standing to avoid pooling of blood. The intensity of your workout should be "somewhat hard," or 12 to 14 on the RPE scale (See Chapter 3.) Be sure to drink water at frequent intervals. Avoid overheating. Stop if you feel any pain or discomfort.

<u>Short cool down</u>

Slow your heart rate down with easy rhythmic leg movements and gentle stretches. It's time to replace some fluids and empty your bladder before starting the body work.

<u>Body work (muscular strength and flexibility)</u>

You work the upper and lower body plus abdominals using smooth and controlled movements. Remember to exhale during the contraction of muscles and inhale during the release. Avoid the supine position for abdominals. Practice good body alignment and body mechanics when changing position.

<u>Final cool down</u>

Combine gentle stretching and relaxation with slow deep breathing. Your pulse rate should be back to normal before you leave class, feeling refreshed and invigorated. "I always feel great after class. I have more energy and feel positive," remarks Julie who is taking a prenatal aerobics class.

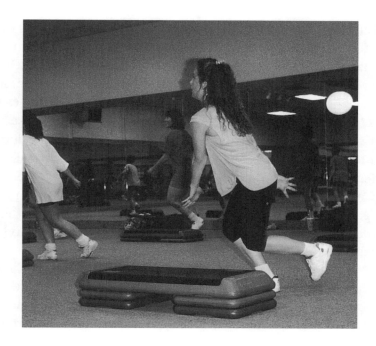

Aerobics movements should be smooth and controlled.

MOMS IN MOTION

Sara Kooperman, JD, an aerobics instructor and owner of Sara's City Workout, Inc. in Chicago, designed Moms in Motion, a prenatal exercise class offered at Northwestern Memorial Hospital. The class was developed to help pregnant women safely exercise during pregnancy, taking into account the tremendous body changes in pregnancy. The following are some of Sara's guidelines for a safe fitness program in pregnancy.

Prior to enrolling in class, all of the students obtain a note of approval from their health care provider. Students are advised to eat a light snack one to two hours before class and to bring a water bottle and towel for floorwork. Sara advises her students to exercise at their own level and to listen to any signals their body might be sending during the workout. The class avoids high impact and power moves (sudden jumps or thrusts) as well as exercises using rubber bands around the ankles. (Some swelling in pregnancy is common so this might cause trauma to the tissue as well as impair circulation.) Likewise, the class avoids any exercises with the head below the heart. (In this position, your expanded blood volume can cause you to feel faint.) Kegel exercises are included in every class to strengthen the pelvic floor muscles. Sara closely observes each student and offers pointers for modifying exercises during each trimester. Time is spent in class talking about pregnancy-related issues like hormonal changes, breast and bottle feeding, baby equipment and other topics. "Participating in Moms In Motion gave me more energy and I had an opportunity to meet other pregnant women," recalls Alison a twenty-six year new mother. "It was a lot of fun."

What if a prenatal aerobics isn't available where you live? One option is to purchase a prenatal exercise videotape. Make sure the tape follows the ACOG guidelines and you take the same precautions as you would if you were participating in an aerobics class. Be sure to exercise in a cool room and drink plenty of fluids.

Another option is to integrate into a regular aerobics class. Discuss this plan with your health care provider. A low impact aerobics class, or bench step class using the platform only with no risers, is safest. Let the instructor know that you are pregnant and closely follow all of the exercise guidelines in pregnancy. Do not try to "keep up" with the class. Instead, exercise at your own pace, paying attention to any signs of discomfort or strain. You may need to eliminate parts of the workout or shorten it all together.

WHEN TO STOP?

You need to stop exercising if you feel any of the following symptoms: Increased uterine contractions, decreased fetal movements, vaginal bleeding, leaking of amniotic fluid, dizziness or faintness, shortness of breath, palpitations, persistent nausea or vomiting, back pain or hip pain, or difficulty walking.

Remember, there's a silent passenger on board, so you need to tune into any signals your body might be sending during your aerobics program.

WHAT OTHERS SAY

The following are some experiences of women who modified their aerobics routines during pregnancy.

Kathy is a 32 year old mother of three and former teacher.
She participated in gymnastics from age seven to thirteen and then
competed in diving during high school. During college she started
attending aerobics classes on a regular basis. While pregnant with
her first two children, she was able to participate in low impact
aerobics three times a week, avoiding abdominals after her fourth
month. In her third pregnancy, she attended a bench step class,
using the platform without risers. She stopped using any hand
weights and did easy arm movements. Kathy felt most comfortable in Spandex shorts and a baggy T-shirt.

In each of her pregnancies, she turned to swimming during the
last two months because of pelvic pressure and varicose veins.
Kathy felt great in the water. With her first pregnancy, because she
was not yet a proficient swimmer, she held a kickboard under her
chest and kicked her way up and down the lap lanes. She swam
until delivery without any major problems. Occasionally, when
climbing out of the pool, she would feel the "pull of gravity" on
her abdomen. After a few seconds, she adjusted to being out of the
buoyant water environment. Kathy monitored herself carefully
during all of her pregnancies and cut back or modified according
to how she felt. "I really enjoyed exercising. I felt it helped me
maintain my shape as much as possible as well as allowed me time
to clear my head." All of Kathy's babies were delivered vaginally and weighed between 7 and 7 3/4 pounds.

"Exercise kept me energized," recalls Alane, a 37 year old
mother of two. Prior to pregnancy Alane taught aerobic dance two
to four hours a week. She continued to teach until her fifth month
when her growing size made it difficult to both instruct the class
and perform the workout. Instead, she attended aerobics 1 to 2
hours a week and began a prenatal water fitness program once a
week. She continued low impact aerobics, making adjustments
for back discomfort by avoiding certain floor exercises, until the

eighth month. "I was concerned about maintaining fitness and tone during pregnancy, but toward the end, I found I concentrated more on flexibility than aerobic exercise." Alane's first labor lasted 19 hours which surprised her. She thought being fit would make her labor easier. No evidence exists in any of the studies that exercise affects the length or quality of labor or lessens the risk of complications. (Mittelmark et al. 1991, p.314) However, being fit helped her to recover and get back in shape more quickly.

7

WEIGHT TRAINING

Walk into any health club and you will see and hear the impact of the weight training industry. The clank of weights and the whirl of cables and pulleys signal that everybody's "using it" so they don't "lose it." There are many good reasons why you too should include weight training in your exercise program. Besides getting stronger, which can enhance athletic performance, you can ward off injuries, build stronger bones, boost your metabolism, feel better about yourself and look great in the process. No wonder the industry is booming!

Weight training is progressive resistance exercise. Free weights (dumbbells and barbells) and exercise machines provide the resistance to the muscles you are working. Resistance stimulates muscle growth as well as improving muscle strength and endurance. You should develop a weight training program that is based on completing certain exercises grouped together by repetitions and sets. Repetitions (reps) are the number of times you do an exercise and sets are the number of groupings of repetitions. Before we look at pregnancy-specific weight training, let's review the basics of a weight training program.

PRINCIPLES OF WEIGHT TRAINING

You should design an individualized weight training program that will meet your goals. Perhaps your goal is to improve your muscular endurance, or maybe it is to build overall strength, or even more likely, to trim and tone as you lose weight. Weight training, when coupled with aerobic exercise and proper diet, can help with weight loss. Aerobic exercise burns calories while lifting weights builds muscles. Bigger muscles burn calories more efficiently (Baechle and Groves, 1992), so it's like cranking up your metabolism. You can achieve all of these goals with a well designed, yet simple, weight training program.

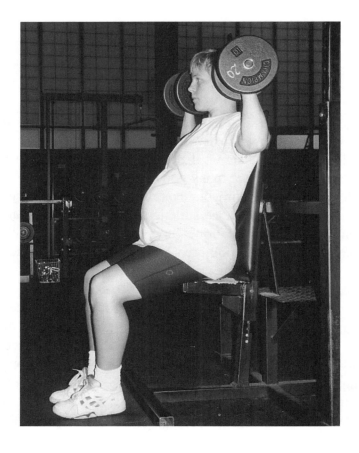

Upper body strength comes in handy after your baby arrives.

Two basic principles, specificity and overload, form the foundation of weight training. Specificity means that you target certain muscle groups in your workout. For example, some women may want to improve their upper body strength. If you are a runner, there's a good chance that you have neglected your upper body strength. A strong upper body helps you maintain good posture, run more efficiently and keep your form. By having a stronger upper body, you'll expend less energy and run farther and faster. Cyclists will want to focus more on strengthening their legs and cross-country skiers want both upper and lower body strength. One thing to keep in mind is this: a strong upper body is every mother's blessing — as you struggle to carry your baby, diaper bag and groceries — all at one time.

The overload principle requires you to progressively increase the intensity of your workout over time in a set pattern. You will do this over a period of weeks and months. Muscles, to get stronger, need to be challenged by slowly increasing the resistance, the number of repetitions, and the rate of work. Using both the specificity and overload concepts, you design a program of weight training which determines the load (amount of weight), the number of reps and sets and the recovery period between the sets.

Trainers, available through health clubs, can help you design your program using these principles. Make sure the person you are working with is qualified and certified by one of these organizations — NSCA (National Strength and Conditioning Association), ACE (American Council on Exercise), ACSM (American College of Sports Medicine). For further information, write to the National Strength and Conditioning Association, P.O. Box 38909, Colorado Springs, CO 80937-6367.

LIFTING FUNDAMENTALS AND EQUIPMENT

Before discussing lifting techniques, let's talk about the importance of a warm-up before your workout and a cool-down afterwards. To avoid injury and help your muscles recover, warm-up with 10 to 15 minutes of brisk walking, jogging, or stationary cycling followed by stretching. This kind of warm-up prepares your muscles and joints for the work ahead. Be sure to include stretches for the chest, shoulders, arms, back and large muscle groups (hamstrings, quadriceps and calves). Don't forget to cool down (easy jogging, walking) and stretch after your workout to prevent muscle soreness. (See Chapter Five for more information.)

Weight training machines are generally safer than free weights. You don't have to worry about weights falling on you nor do you need the help of a "spotter," someone who assists you in performing a particular lift. Become familiar with the machines at your facility. If you are not sure about a particular machine — ask.

- Adjust levers and seats to comfortable positions. (These may change during your pregnancy.)
- Avoid bouncing the weight stacks.
- Perform each exercise slowly and with control, using a full range of motion.
- Load the bars evenly.
- Properly lock the barbells and dumbbells — don't assume the person ahead of you did.
- Be aware of other lifters around you — pay attention!
- Replace and store the equipment you use.

Technique

Proper technique is very important whether you are using free weights or weight machines. You cannot only avoid injuries to muscles, tendons and bones, you can get better results.

Correct lifting

Use a light grip — not a "death" grip. The focus of your energy should be on the muscles you are working rather than your hands. Lift from a stable position. Keep the weight close to your body.

Breathing

Whether using weight machines or free weights, you always want to breathe out (exhale) during the lifting or exertion phase and breathe in (inhale) during the recovery or lowering phase. During pregnancy, avoid the Valsalva maneuver (holding your breath while lifting or moving a weight). Holding your breath while lifting can raise your blood pressure and decrease blood flow to the uterus.

Spotters

Some lifts require spotters, someone who is ready to assist you as you perform lifts like the bench press. During your pregnancy it is best to avoid the lifts that require a spotter. There are safer alternative exercises you can do with weight machines.

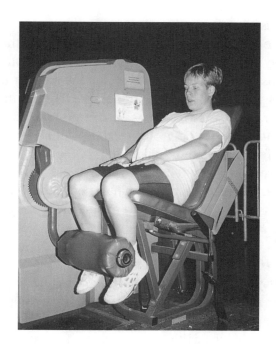

Wear comfortable clothing. A large T shirt
over cycling-style shorts or tights works well.

I am assuming that you have worked with a trainer to set up a weight training program and that you have already determined your training loads for each exercise. A training load is a set weight that allows you to do up to 12 reps (repetitions) of that particular exercise. With each rep, use slow controlled movements, a full range of motion, and proper breathing techniques. (Exhale with the lift, inhale with the recovery.) For best results, try to weight train two to three days a week, with a recovery day after each session.

Your program should work all the muscle groups — chest, arms, shoulders, back, thighs and abdomen. Try to:

1. Work all the large muscles first.
2. Alternate push with pull exercises.
3. Alternate upper body with lower body exercises.
4. Work opposing muscle groups i.e., biceps/triceps, quads/hamstrings, etc.

Tailor your program around the training loads, the number of reps (usually 8-12), the number of sets (the times you perform the block of reps — usually 2 to 3 sets), and the rest periods between each set. As you get stronger, you increase the training loads.

If you are pressed for time, you can do split routines which allows you to work for a shorter period of time on specific body parts on different days. For example, in a four day per week program, two workouts would focus on your upper body (chest, shoulders, triceps, biceps, upper abdominal, upper back) and the other two workouts would concentrate on your lower body (legs, lower back, lower abdominal).

PREGNANCY WEIGHT TRAINING

Most of you will find that you can continue weight training during your pregnancy as long as you modify your routine and take some basic precautions. As with any exercise activity, be sure to consult with your health care provider if there are any special concerns about your pregnancy or general health. Stick with weight machines unless you are experienced with free weights. Now, more than ever, you need to practice good technique and follow all the lifting fundamentals. Here are some important points to consider.

Warm-up/Cooldown

As mentioned earlier, pregnancy relaxes your joints and ligaments. Proper warm-up and cool down will prevent injury.

Fluids

Carry a water bottle with you on your circuit and drink often.

Clothing

Wear comfortable clothing. A large T shirt over cycling-style shorts or tights works well. Stay cool. Don't overdress. Supportive running or aerobic shoes are fine for the feet.

EXERCISES TO AVOID

After the first trimester, you should avoid exercises which require you to lie on your back (supine position) or stomach. You can still work these muscles in a more upright position. For example, for the chest, instead of the free weight bench press or dumbbell flys, you can substitute the bent arm fly using a "pec dec" chest machine. This machine can approximate the fly movement and works your pectoral (chest) muscles. For your back, use the cam rowing machine or the seated rowing exercise instead of the barbell bent-over row exercise.

Avoid power lifting and quick-lift exercises. Power lifting is a sport that develops maximum strength using specific lifts. Quick-lifts require explosive movements. Do neither of these techniques during your pregnancy. If you body build, discuss this with your health provider.

PRACTICE SAFE LIFTING TECHNIQUES

As your pregnancy continues and you get bigger, your center of gravity will shift. Pay attention to your body position as you perform your exercise circuit. Use good body mechanics as you load weight machines with weights. Your lower back is vulnerable to injury as well as joints and ligaments. Working with a friend or partner is fun. Then, you can converse as you lift, which helps keep your heart rate down, and you will have someone to observe your technique. Your partner can also remind you to breathe correctly — to exhale with the lift, inhale on recovery.

MODIFY MODIFY MODIFY

As your body changes over the next nine months, so will your weight training program. Switch to lighter weights and moderate repetitions. Extend your recovery phase in-between exercises. Always work under the supervision of your health care provider and a trained fitness instructor. Listen to your body. You are weight training to maintain tone and fitness — not to re-sculpture your body or train for power lifting. Stop if you feel faint, short of breath, or experience any pain or bleeding.

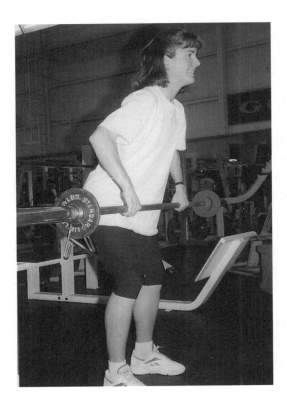

Instead of barbell
bent rows ...

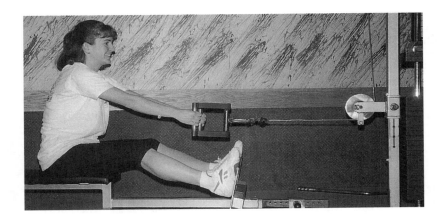

....substitute seated rowing.

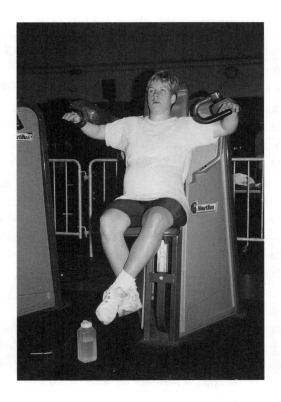

Carry a water bottle with you on your circuit and drink often.

SHANNON'S PROGRAM

During high school Shannon played volleyball and softball and ran cross-country. When she entered college, she began weight training to improve her overall strength and endurance. Her studies in exercise science helped her to design a program to achieve these goals. As her fitness and strength improved, so did her commitment to her weight training program. When she finished college she took a position as a fitness coordinator at a university fitness and wellness center. At this point, her program consisted of twenty minutes of aerobic exercise (Stairmaster) followed by 1 to 1 1/2 hours of weight training three to six days a week using both free weights and weight machines.

When Shannon, who was now 23, learned she was pregnant, she wanted to continue her program with some modifications. At her first prenatal visit, accompanied by her husband, she discussed her current fitness program with her health care provider. Together, they agreed that the health of her pregnancy was the number one priority and that her new fitness goal was to maintain her fitness and not to improve on strength and endurance. Shannon and her health provider reviewed the exercise guidelines for pregnancy. (See Chapter 3).

Her program remained the same during her first trimester though now she made sure she ate a light snack an hour before her workout and drank plenty of water. Plagued by some nausea and fatigue, she found that exercising helped relieve these symptoms. By the second trimester she eliminated any lifting on her back or stomach and cut back on her workouts. Shannon gradually decreased the weights and increased the reps to the 12 to 15 range. "I always listened to my body and was extremely cautious. I stopped if anything felt sore or uncomfortable. My husband was very supportive as was everyone else at the fitness center." By the time Shannon went into labor she had gained about 24 pounds. During her labor, the fetus' heart rate pattern was showing signs of distress. A healthy baby boy, "Cyrus," was delivered by Cesarean section and weighed in at nine pounds, one ounce. "I think being in shape helped give me the stamina to tolerate labor better, and it certainly has helped me with recovery after the surgery. I hope to slowly get back to my program."

Shannon's story is a good lesson: exercise does not guarantee the elimination of complications during pregnancy and delivery. Yet it is important to keep in mind that you and your baby are still ahead of the game in spite of one or two setbacks.

8

RUNNING AND WALKING

RUNNING

The beauty of running is its simplicity. Strap on a pair of running shoes, find a road or trail, and you are ready for an invigorating cardiovascular workout. When running outdoors, it's fun to treat your senses to the sights, smells and sounds of your route, letting the fresh mown grass, the colorful leaves, or the crunching snow remind you of the changing seasons. It's little wonder that running is one of today's most popular fitness activities.

Running is a time-efficient aerobic activity. You can squeeze a workout into a lunch hour, go out before breakfast, or tag a run on at the end of the day. Even with a busy schedule, you can usually find time for a run — something to keep in mind, especially after you have the baby and time is precious.

If you already run, you will likely want to continue it during pregnancy. In general, running is a safe activity that many pregnant women continue, with modification, throughout pregnancy. If you've never run before, now is not the time to start. If you are a seasoned runner, you'll enjoy the journey ahead.

Several studies have looked at the safety of running in pregnancy. In 1981 the Melpomene Institute, a non-profit organization which publishes research and educational material on fitness and health for girls and women, completed a study on pregnant runners. (Melpomene Institute 1990) One hundred ninety-five women, whose average age was 29.1 years, were studied. Three months before conception they were averaging 24.8 miles per week. 80.3% of the women delivered vaginally while 19.7% had Cesarean sections. The average birth weight was seven pounds, six ounces. All the infants were born healthy and survived the neonatal period. This report and other studies (Hauth et al. 1982; Jarret and Spellacy 1983) on pregnant runners are reassuring. You can continue to run as long as you follow some special guidelines.

STARTING THE RUN
If you're the type who laces up your shoes and then bounds out the door without stretching, change your ways! Now that you're carrying a future runner, you need to take some extra precautions. More than ever, proper stretching both before and after running, will help prevent injuries. Relaxin, the hormone that relaxes your ligaments, is working throughout pregnancy. Loose joints and ligaments make you more vulnerable to injury so concentrate on stretches for your large muscles ... hamstrings, quadriceps, calf muscles, Achilles and lower back muscles (Mittelmark et al., 1991 p 123, 131). Gentle, easy stretching is best. (See Chapter 5 for specific stretches and cool downs.) Sip some water as you stretch. Listening to some music may help cut the boredom and encourage you to warm up adequately. Hit the bathroom one last time and start out slowly.

Follow a few simple rules to make your run more enjoyable and safer. First, if you're running alone, let someone know your route and the approximate time you'll be back. I suggest that you run with a buddy — it is safer and keeps your workout intensity at the "talk test" level. (You should be able to carry on a conversation as you run.) Second, carry spare change in case you need to make an emergency phone call and always carry some form of identification as well. Third, wear reflective clothing or vests at dawn or dusk or whenever the visibility is low. Finally, leave your Sony Walkman™ at home. Your attention needs to be on you and the road.

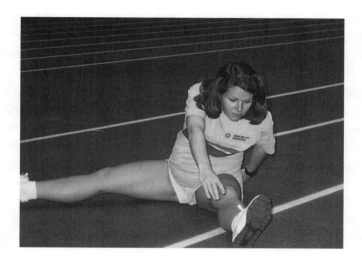

Now, more than ever, proper stretching both before and after running, will help prevent injuries.

LISTEN TO YOUR BODY

You will need to modify the intensity, frequency, and speed of your runs. Remember, you are running to maintain your fitness, not to train. Slow down — don't push your pace, and don't push your distance. Back off running a preset course if you just don't feel like doing it.

Stop and walk if you feel Braxton Hicks contractions (rhythmic tightenings of the lower abdomen) or ligament pains. At seven months, I sometimes felt Braxton Hicks contractions during the first few minutes of a run. I would stop and walk for a few minutes and then, when the contractions stopped, start up again slowly.

Stop if you feel pain, persistent contractions, leakage of fluid, fatigue, dizziness, or any other medical problem.

WHERE TO RUN?

Most of you are probably road rats and have several favorite running routes. During pregnancy, you can probably still run most of them if you keep several things in mind:

- Pick a route with a phone and bathroom facility nearby.
- For safety, avoid country roads with long, open stretches.
- Stay off roads with rough, uneven pavement. You don't want to spend most of your concentration and energy dodging potholes and wobbling along on narrow, fractured road shoulders.
- Skip routes with steep hills. Uphills may push your intensity level too high. Downhills put a lot of stress on knees and can, due to your extra weight and relaxed joints, cause knee injuries.

Running on an outdoor track may sound boring to some of you and painfully familiar to others. But, when you're pregnant, you will find the overall the smooth, softer surface kinder to your changing body — and there are usually bathrooms nearby.

Weather conditions will also determine where you run. Snow and ice can make running extremely dangerous — even more so when you are a little top heavy with your pregnancy. Winters in Central New York where I live are notorious for persistent snow, and we get used to running on snow-covered roads and sidewalks. Hours before a major record snow storm, I saw our neighbor, nine months pregnant, "jogging" in nearly a foot of snow. When I talked to her later, she admitted that it would have been safer to bag the run and do an indoor workout. When the weather is lousy, move your workout inside. If you have use of an indoor track — great! Other options are a stationary bike, a treadmill, a NordicTrack,™ or an aerobics tape.

WHAT TO WEAR?

Early in pregnancy, your regular running attire will work fine. As your abdomen begins to expand, you will need clothes that provide comfort and support.

First, let's look at comfort. Wear running gear that is comfortable and doesn't bind. Finally, a good use for all those large race T-shirts! Spandex cycling shorts or tights will stretch as you grow. You may like the added snugness and longer lengths. I know I did.

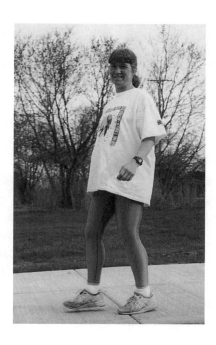

Wear running gear that is comfortable and doesn't bind.

During the last few months of my pregnancy, I liked wearing a prenatal abdominal support. Even though I was not carrying the pregnancy low, the added support to my lower abdomen felt good. Abdominal support gear comes in different styles and sizes. If you have varicose veins, running in maternity support hose offers some additional support. As I mentioned in Chapter 2, sport bras or supportive bras with wide straps are more comfortable for running.

Dress for the weather. Wear light loose fitting clothing in warmer weather. As we noted in Chapter 3, staying cool is important. Avoid running in hazy, hot and humid weather. In cooler weather, dress in layers. You may find that you sweat more when pregnant so check out the new moisture wicking fabrics which will help keep you drier. Protect your extremities when running in the cold. Wear a hat to avoid heat loss off your head as well as warm mittens and gloves. When it's cold, overdress. You can always peel off layers as you go along.

SHOES

Let's take a look at your shoes. You know your feet better than anyone, so the brand and model you're running in now probably works fine. During your pregnancy however, you need to consider a few things about your feet and your running shoes.

Your feet will be supporting a lot more of you in the next nine months. Normally, when running, you land with an impact three times your body weight. Your feet, specifically your heels, will be bearing the brunt of the impact. Put your lighter racing flats away for now. You'll need a shoe with at least 3/4 inch cushioning in the heel. Expect your feet to swell, which can increase your shoe size by a half size. Compensate by wearing a shoe with a wide toe box. Shop for a new pair of running shoes in the afternoon when your feet are apt to be swollen. Buy what feels comfortable. While you are at it, pick up a pair of lace locks — instead of lacing your shoes, you slide the laces through a small plastic device that secures the lace. It sure beats bending over and tying the laces.

The socks you wear should be smooth fitting and conform to your feet. Swelling and sweating — the woes of "pregnant feet" — will feel better in light synthetic materials that wick away moisture and prevent blisters.

RUNNING IN EARLY PREGNANCY

You may experience bouts of nausea and fatigue the first few months. Several runners that I interviewed found that running in the morning helped. An elite runner stated: "As soon as I go out to run, it's strange, but it [nausea] is almost immediately gone." Another runner agrees: "After my morning run, my morning sickness always went away."

Try running outdoors if you normally run on an indoor track. The fresh air may help. If you find yourself losing weight from vomiting, cut back your running or stop until you are gaining adequate weight. Talk to your health provider about it.

Fatigue can be perplexing these first few months. As an active woman, you are used to feeling energetic most of the time. Before pregnancy, if you felt sluggish, you probably went out for a run to regain some vigor. Now you may be more inclined to curl up for a nap. The fatigue of early pregnancy can feel as if you're under the influence of a sleeping pill. One woman put it like this, "I felt like I could sleep all day even after an eight hour sleep."

Schedule your run at a time of day when you feel least tired. Don't push it. It can be frustrating — in your mind, you know that running will probably make you feel better, but your body is saying "doze." If running seems too much for today, substitute a brisk walk, a few laps in the pool, or spinning on a stationary bike. Be flexible and patient. The advice to remember: "This too shall pass."

As mentioned earlier, running with tender swollen breasts is uncomfortable. "It was the least pleasant pregnancy change for me," recalled an elite runner. Buy a good supportive bra with wide adjustable straps or a sports bra. As weeks go by, you may need to move up to a larger size.

Urinary frequency, one of the early signs of pregnancy, is a challenge. (It also returns later in pregnancy because of the added weight and pressure on your bladder.) For running, you need to devise some strategic plans. Don't cut back on your fluids ... you need to stay well hydrated. Plan your runs around a bathroom stop. A twice-around loop that includes a "pit stop" is one solution. Consider wearing a panty liner just in case.

As you can see, it's important to tailor your running to how you feel and the health of your pregnancy these first few months. Be sure to immediately stop any racing, speed work, or vigorous long runs once you learn that you are pregnant. Keep your workouts in the "somewhat hard range" in the Rate of Perceived Exertion scale. (See Chapter 3)

RUNNING IN LATER PREGNANCY

"I felt the strongest, lots of energy ... no morning sickness," recalls a world class runner about the second trimester of her pregnancy. Yes, it's true, at midpoint (four to seven months) you may feel your best, but you'll also be aware of the added weight and minor aches and pains. It is time to slow down, decrease your mileage, and consider some running alternatives.

Most women I interviewed cut back their mileage 30 to 40% by the second trimester and up to 70% in the last weeks. Some women stopped running altogether because of the extra weight and abdominal pressure. Your running gait changes so be alert to terrain and traffic. You tend to not pick your feet up as high and your stride shortens.

I used to day-dream while running. I would think about the growing being inside me or sort through baby names in my mind until loose pavement or an oncoming car would get me back in focus. I learned to stay alert and run cautiously.

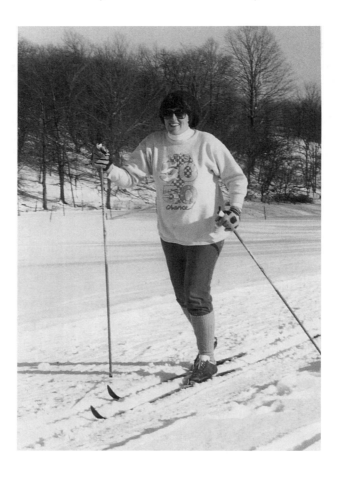

If running becomes uncomfortable, consider non-jarring options.

If running becomes uncomfortable, consider non-weight bearing options for exercise. As a runner, you've probably already engaged in cross-training activities. If you are planning a pregnancy and run exclusively, now, before conception, is the time to introduce yourself to some other activities. In other parts of this book, you can review such options as swimming, paddling, cycling, cross country skiing, Nordic track, low impact aerobics, and walking. Find activities that you can safely enjoy throughout pregnancy.

WALKING

Walking is a good safe alternative throughout your pregnancy. It is less jarring and puts less stress on your ligaments and joints. If done using correct form and with purpose, walking can be just as invigorating as running and a welcome change.

Sore ligaments, pelvic pressure, Braxton Hicks contractions and urinary frequency are common "end stage" complaints and force many women to cut back or cease running. Substituting walking for running or alternating running and walking is a great way to move through the later part of pregnancy. Unless a medical problem intervenes, make your own decision as to when to cutback or stop your running.

One of the great things about walking is that you and your partner can share this activity, as well as some conversation, without the stress of trying to keep up with each other. Later, while pushing a baby stroller you will be "strolling," but now, during your pregnancy, you will most likely be walking briskly at an 18 to 14 minute per mile pace. Here are some tips to consider:

- Shoes. You may want to buy a shoe specifically designed for walking if you plan to walk a lot. A walking shoe has a lower heel (1/2 inch) versus a running shoe which is usually 3/4 inch. A lower, more firm heel is less tiring for walking.
- Walking gait. Like your running gait, your walking gait is also altered in the later months of your pregnancy. When walking briskly, you need to pay attention to your posture and arm and leg swing. Keep your head straight with your chin parallel to the ground. Keep your head up and looking forward. Your shoulders need to be looseand level. Try to keep your hips

under your shoulders avoiding a sway back. Your stride length should be what normally feels comfortable.

- Arm swing. Just like in running, your arms play an important role in helping you move faster and more efficiently. The arms counterbalance and complement your legs as you move. Bend your arm at the elbow so it forms a 90 degree angle. Keep your elbow locked as you swing it toward the front stopping as the hand just reaches the center of your chest. Swing it back until it reaches just about mid-buttocks. Put some force and power in your arm swing. Forget arm and leg weights — they alter your normal arm and leg swing and may cause injury. Besides, you're carrying enough added weight.

HIKING

Hiking is a pleasurable activity you can enjoy throughout your pregnancy. Day hikes with your partner or friends provide an opportunity to explore nature while getting some exercise. Hiking is also an activity you can continue later on with your baby in a carrier or with young children for short outings.

As with any sport or activity, you need to dress for the weather, especially if you will be changing elevation. Layer your clothing or carry extra gear in a backpack along with snacks and water. The newer, lightweight hiking shoes (manufactured by many running shoe companies) are comfortable and durable. You need the higher boot for added support if you are hiking any distance or over changing terrain. Remember, your joints and ligaments (especially your ankles in this case) are vulnerable to strains or sprains. Comfortable socks with extra padding will prevent friction and blisters.

Use common sense. Avoid rugged terrain, "bushwhacking," steep ascents or slick conditions. Stick with familiar trails or ones you have mapped out carefully. County, state, or national parks often have well-marked trails as well as bathroom facilities. You should not hike at altitudes over 8,000 feet due to the decrease in oxygen at higher elevations. Regardless of the altitude, keep a safe comfortable pace with frequent rest and water stops. The fresh air, the solitude, and the slower pace provide an opportunity to move with your thoughts while getting some exercise.

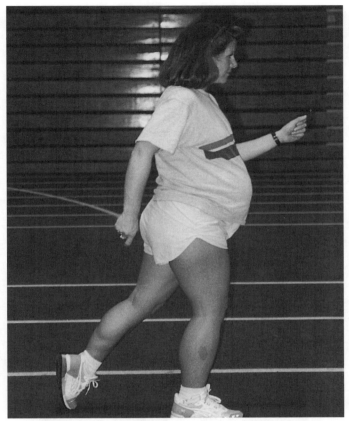

Put some force into your arm swing while walking.

PERSONAL EXPERIENCES

Mary, a thirty-seven year old runner and competitor ran approximately thirty miles a week before pregnancy. During the first trimester she continued to run. A thyroid problem developed during her second trimester which left her with little energy. Under her doctor's guidance, while taking thyroid medication, she was able to walk vigorously several times a week and occasionally swim. She did daily stretching exercises to maintain her flexibility. She delivered a six pound, five ounce healthy baby girl after an eight hour labor. Though she missed running, when she did exercise, she felt "invigorated" and "healthier."

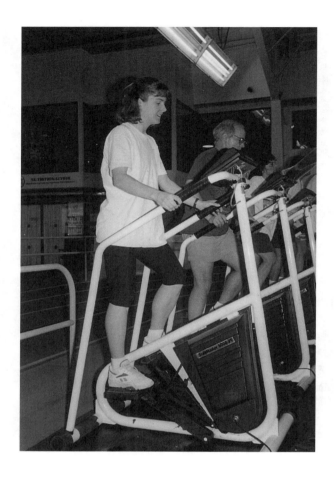

Find activities that you can safely enjoy throughout pregnancy.

Linda, a thirty-four year old mother of two, maintained a running schedule during her pregnancies averaging about thirty to thirty-five miles a week. In the first and second trimesters, she ran the same distance but slowed her pace. During the third trimester she ran half as much and supplemented by walking. The added weight and winter conditions made it difficult to continue running the same distance. Linda, like many women I spoke with, felt positive about feeling "fit" during her pregnancies and benefited from the stress reduction of daily exercise.

A former Alpine ski racer, Carol, pursued a variety of athletic activities before her three pregnancies. She raced canoes, competed in triathlons (swimming, cycling and running or running, cycling and paddling in a canoe) and cross country skied. She ran and cross country skied throughout all of her pregnancies. For two of her pregnancies, she participated in a study on exercise in pregnancy. "The support system of both the other study participants and the research doctor helped me to better understand my changing body and encouraged me to continue running."

"I felt that it was the best thing for me and my baby," Karen, a thirty one year old mother of two said when she described the program of low impact aerobics, Stairmaster' and walking she used during her last pregnancy. During the last two months before delivery, she did more walking due to discomfort from varicose veins. Her second baby was a vaginal delivery after a prior Cesarean section (VBAC). She attributes her stamina during labor and delivery to her exercise program during pregnancy.

A world class runner didn't think of herself as an "athlete" while pregnant. Instead she looked at her pregnancy as though she were "in training" for pregnancy and delivery of a healthy baby. She cut back her running from 70 miles a week to 4 to 5 easy miles a day. In the final weeks she reduced this to 1.5 to 2 miles a day. Sometimes she rode her bike while her husband, an Olympic marathoner, ran. She delivered a six and a half pound healthy baby.

Mary Anne ran during both her pregnancies. "I no longer ran for time. I would cut back immediately if I felt tired." She reduced her mileage each trimester and walked 3 to 4 miles a day the last six weeks because of what she described as shin discomfort. Though never diagnosed, it is likely that her anterolateral leg pain was due to swelling and distention of the fascia, the thin connective tissue, which covers the lower leg muscles. Walking was a wise alternative to running. After an hour and a half labor, Mary Anne had a healthy seven pound, six ounce boy.

At thirty-seven, Barbara became pregnant with her second child. She had been running 8 to 10 miles a week plus weight training mixed in with occasional aerobics classes and stationary cycling. During her second trimester, she cut back on the aerobics and ran more but at a much slower pace. "Even with the extra weight, I enjoyed passing people on the track who were less fit than me. It helps to keep it fun when I feel I'm barely moving sometimes." She successfully delivered a seven pound, eleven ounce boy vaginally, after a previous Cesarean section (VBAC).

Kathleen, a nationally ranked runner and physical therapist, ran during her first pregnancy. While she did not run competitively, during the first two trimesters she rotated "hard" and "easy" days for her runs. Like another competitive runner, Kathleen felt that her morning runs help to eliminate morning sickness, "It's strange, but as soon as I go out to run, it (nausea) is almost immediately gone." The last trimester was all easy running except for the last two weeks when she walked daily. Her labor lasted thirty-six hours. She feels that being in shape helped to provide the stamina to deliver a healthy eight pound, ten ounce baby. Three to four months after her first delivery she ran a 10k race in close to 35 minutes. She recently had her second baby who weighed in at seven pound, three ounces. She ran during this pregnancy, sometimes using a baby jogger. She says, "Most people who exercise regularly are in touch with their bodies...all you need to do is listen to yours and make adjustments accordingly."

Kathleen speaks for many fit moms when she told me, "Exercise is wonderful!"

9

Swimming and Water Activities

SWIMMING

I spent some of my most pleasurable memories during pregnancy submerged in water staring at a blue line at the bottom of a swimming pool. My view rolled with each stroke, one moment the lit pool room and the next moment the blue line below as I rhythmically breathed with each stroke. The water buoyed my expanding abdomen — I felt less big — less awkward — less pregnant! No doubt about it, swimming felt great!

I usually swam in the morning which helped lessen my bouts with nausea and gave me more energy for working during the day. In the water, my mind would wander to thoughts of the baby inside — imagining what he or she might be feeling as we rhythmically moved through the water. The baby tended to be less active during these early morning workouts. "Probably napping," I thought.

If you swam as a fitness activity before you became pregnant, there's an excellent chance you will be able to continue from conception right up to the delivery of your baby. "I stopped the day before my baby was born," reported an experienced swimmer who swam throughout her pregnancy. Another, who did the same, said, "I finished swimming one hour before my labor began. During early labor you may even find yourself submerged in water in a tub at your hospital or birthing center. Warm water is a great muscle relaxer and pain reliever.

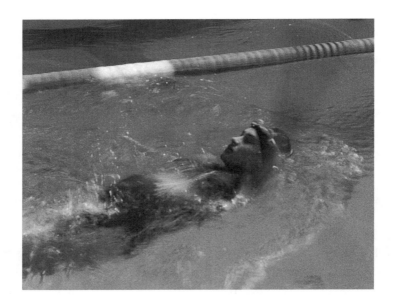

The water surrounding your body keeps you cool while exercising.

If you are planning pregnancy in the future, now would be a good time to brush up on your swimming technique. Swimming may end up being the one exercise that will get you through the last lap of pregnancy. If you are a scuba diver, retire your wet suit and tank during preganancy — the risks to the fetus in a submerged environment are not known at this point.

As mentioned previously, the hormones of pregnancy relax your joints and ligaments making them vulnerable to injury. The buoyancy of water provides you with a gentle buffer against strain and injury. Swimming helps you build endurance and strengthen and tone your muscles, especially your arms and legs. When you are submerged in water, fluid in your tissues is forced back into your bloodstream. This process helps reduce swelling, a common problem later in pregnancy. Pregnant swimmers notice more of an urge to empty their bladders. This is the way your body gets rid of the extra fluid so be sure to empty your bladder right before a swim and be prepared to take a bathroom break. One thirty-seven year old mother who swam five days a week, stated, "Swimming kept me toned, and I had no water retention at all."

You are less likely to overheat while swimming because the water surrounding your body keeps you cool while exercising. The rhythmic breathing in swimming is great practice for relaxed breathing during your labor. Try visualizing your labor while doing laps and maintaining a rhythmic pattern of slow, deep breathing. Stay relaxed and focused. One thirty-two year old swimmer summed it like this, "Swimming helped me prepare for the intensity of labor. It helped me to cope with the physical demands of labor much better."

INTO THE POOL

Before continuing your swim program, discuss your plans with your health care provider. Let him or her know how often and how long you are swimming, at what intensity, and how you are feeling as your pregnancy progresses. Remember, you are swimming to maintain your fitness, not to train or compete. This is a time to tune into your body and listen to any signals it might be sending.

What to wear?

Maternity swim suits create more drag because of the extra material that acts as a "cover up." You will probably be more comfortable in a nylon or lycra one piece suit, a size or two larger. Besides, why "hide" your pregnancy? A sports bra worn underneath will help give extra support and reduce breast tenderness. "I wore my old stretched out suits, some 'junk' suits from a friend and bought one suit in a bigger size," one swimmer told me. A swim cap keeps your hair out of your eyes and helps protect your hair against the damage of chlorine. Special shampoos to eliminate chlorine are a good idea. Goggles protect your eyes from irritation and improve your vision.

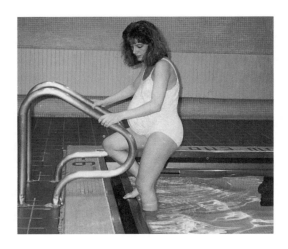

For safety's sake, don't dive after the first trimester.

Ready — Set — Go!

The temperature of the pool should be between 83 and 86 degrees (Mittelmark et al. 1991, p. 272). Warmer temperatures may cause overheating and cooler temperatures will cause excessive heat loss and shivering. Schedule your swim when the pool is least crowded. Sharing a lane with a "lane hog" can be frustrating and potentially dangerous. You also end up focusing more attention on the other swimmer which takes away the enjoyment of your swim.

Before getting into the pool, empty your bladder and do a few stretches for your arms and legs. Avoid jumping into the pool feet first due to the rare possibility of water being forced into your vagina. For safety's sake, don't dive after the first trimester. Start off slowly and gradually pick up your pace after you are warmed up. Always swim in a supervised pool or if you are swimming in a lake, with a buddy.

Most of you can continue to do all swim strokes — freestyle (crawl), backstroke, and breaststroke — that you normally use for workouts. More experienced swimmers can still do the butterfly — which requires more energy and technique. Whatever stroke you use, concentrate on good form and stroke technique to move your changing body efficiently through the water. Keep your strokes long and relaxed. Try to get as much distance as possible with each stroke. Just as in other sports, it's safest to eliminate speedwork and competition unless you are an elite swimmer under the guidance of a health care professional.

Freestyle

For the freestyle stroke, your palms should be facing your feet with each stroke. Your hands, not your elbows, lead the pull of the stroke. Keep the waterline at your hairline. When breathing, allow your head to move independently of your upper body. Lift and turn your head with your neck. As soon as you take a quick breath, return to the face down position. The underwater arm pull in the freestyle is an elongated "S," with the elbow bent, up to 90 degrees. Keep your elbow high and your forearm relaxed. Your hand enters the water at a 45 degree angle in front of your shoulders.

In later pregnancy, your expanding abdomen will create more drag (resistance) in the water. The tendency will be for you to kick harder using up more energy. Keep your kicks small and moderate or consider wearing fins to give you more propulsion. Relax your ankles and bend your knees slightly on the downbeat, straightening them on the upbeat. Only your heels should break the surface.

Breaststroke

Relaxation in your hips and pelvis from the hormones of pregnancy make the frog kick of the breaststroke uncomfortable. Try slowing down your kick and keep your knees closer together. Leslie, an experienced swimmer, as well as other swimmers I spoke with, felt soreness in their lower backs during the breaststroke. Posture adjustments in pregnancy cause an increase in the curvature of your lower spine. The breaststroke may exacerbate this problem.

Backstroke

Some women I spoke with felt fine doing the backstroke in later pregnancy while others felt more awkward. The profile of your abdomen cruising through the water will certainly be an eye opener at your pool. "I felt less coordinated on my back. It was hard to keep good form with the added heaviness of my abdomen," remarked Karen at eight months. She stuck with the freestyle and breaststroke during the remainder of her pregnancy.

Choose the strokes that feel most comfortable for you and be willing to modify according to how you feel on any given day. What about flip turns? Most women eliminate these as they get bigger. One told me, "It was harder for me to get into a tuck for flip turns near the end of my pregnancy. It was more important for me to keep a steady pace during my swims." She also noted that she had to resort to using the ladder to get in and out of the pool — definitely "un-cool," in her words, since "real" swimmers make their exits out of the water on their arms.

<u>Training Devices</u>

Training devices can add some fun and focus to your pool swims. Pull buoys, a flotation device placed between your legs, keeps your lower body buoyant while you concentrate on your arm stroke. Lisa, a triathlete, used a pull buoy to match the buoyancy of her growing abdomen. She found that her legs tended to sink without the pull buoy.

Hand paddles come in various sizes and help strengthen your shoulders, chest and back. The added resistance makes your upper body work harder. If you haven't used these before pregnancy, don't start now. They require good technique and might cause injury if not used properly.

A kickboard allows you to build leg strength and concentrate on your kick. Kathy, a mother of three, used a kickboard for swimming during her second pregnancy. At the time, she was not a strong swimmer so she placed the board under her chest for added buoyancy and proceeded to do lap after lap, kicking all the way! You can use a kickboard to break up your swim and strengthen your lower body. A few swimmers I spoke with noticed a jump in their heart rates while kicking with a board. Your heart has to work harder to pump oxygen to your working leg muscles. Slow the kick down and rest longer between laps.

Swim fins help you develop ankle flexibility and stroke technique. The propulsion of the fins provides stability and balance. Fins can help you overcome the added drag of your growing abdomen and still maintain good form. It's a great feeling to cruise along as your feet flutter effortlessly. Try them and enjoy the ride!

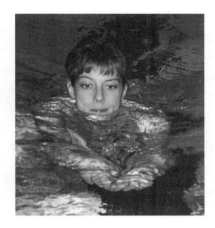

The breastroke

The sidestroke

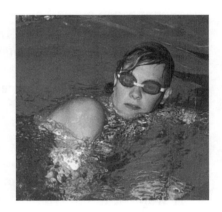

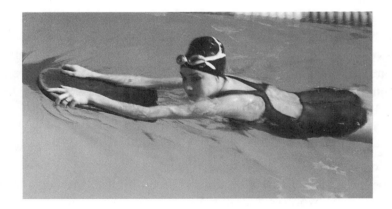

A kickboard lets you to build leg strength and concentrate on your kick.

WATER EXERCISE

Water aerobics and water exercise, like swimming, use the buoyancy and resistance of water for a beneficial, non-weight bearing workout. The buoyancy of the water prevents jarring and jerky movements and puts less strain on your limbs and joints. At the same time, the resistance of the water helps you build strength, endurance and flexibility.

You can find water aerobics classes at many YWCA's, community pools, and health clubs. Check to see if there is a special prenatal water aerobics class in your area. Wear a comfortable suit with a supportive bra. If you wear glasses, stabilize them with a head band before getting in the water. Movements in the water are choreographed to music. (A boom box really bangs it out in a pool room — your baby will love it!) Use a full range of motion with slower, yet forceful movements for your arms and legs. Bigger movements push more water, giving you a better workout. Sometimes hand held devices like paddles or jugs are used to create more resistance when working the arms and shoulder muscles. Keep your breathing even. Be aware of any signs of strain. Stop or modify the movement if you feel discomfort or pain. You should be able to carry on a conversation or sing along with the music during your workout. Keep your intensity level moderate.

A workout in the pool keeps your heart rate lower than the same workout on land (Mittlemark et al., 1991, p. 274). The physiological effects of being submerged in water is responsible for this "user-friendly" response. Exercising in water keeps you cooler and prevents overheating. However, you still need to drink plenty of water before and after your workout. Classes end with gentle stretching to bring your heart rate down and relax your muscles.

If a water aerobics class is not available where you live, you can use the pool for some water calisthenics or walking and jogging in place. Flotation belts or vests keep you vertical for walking or jogging. Design your own water workout — let those creative juices flow! Use a kickboard or hold on to the edge of the pool for leg work or kicking. Work both your lower and upper body. Keep the movements big and make sure your breathing is slow and relaxed. End your workout with some gentle stretching.

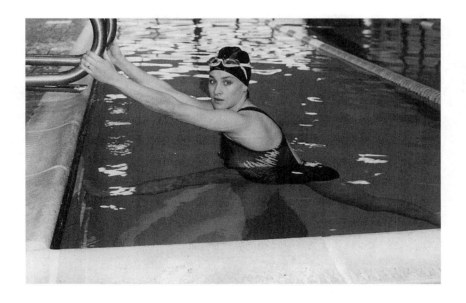

Use the side of the pool and design your own water workout.

CANOEING AND ROWING

Being in the water feels terrific while you are pregnant, but so does being on the water. Paddling a canoe or rowing in a shell are two non-impact aerobic activities that translate well into the physiological changes of pregnancy. Your weight is supported by the canoe or shell so there is little risk of injury to your joints or ligaments from heavy impact. Either activity gets you outdoors where you can savor the peace and beauty of a lake or river.

Living near a lake has provided me with many pleasurable early morning paddles on clear, calm waters. The simple task of thrusting a paddle into water and powering the movement of a sleek Kevlar canoe is my version of a great wake-up call. I try to get out shortly after sunrise when sometimes I meet a lone fishing boat or a covey of ducks on the journey up the west side of the lake. I gaze ahead at the bow of the canoe and watch the water being displaced by the power of my efforts. By the turnaround, the wind has picked up, and now, with the wind at my back, I head

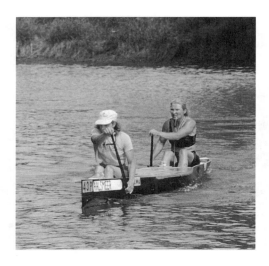

Elite female paddlers have upper body strength that is
proportional to their bodies and are cardiovascularly fit.

home. I struggle to stay flat and keep a straight course. Once at
the shoreline, I pause, and sit in the canoe and gaze at the still-
quiet lake. I paddled right up to delivery, always enjoying a re-
freshing morning workout.

Paddling a canoe is a sport open to women of all ages and
athletic backgrounds, from the recreational paddler to the serious
competitor. Women are well suited for canoe racing. You don't
have to have bulky biceps or a chest like Godzilla to power a canoe. Most of the power comes from your back and torso. When
you think about it, your physical efforts push your canoe and the
weight of your body through water. Elite female paddlers have
upper body strength that is proportional to their bodies and are
cardiovascularly fit. These women have mastered the skills and
techniques of canoe racing and have the strength and determination to go the distance.

For recreational purposes, a standard canoe made of aluminum or fiberglass fits the bill. Serious competitors move up to
sleek racing canoes. Competition cruisers (C-2) have swept-in bows
and sterns and are built to go fast. The design may vary depending

on the weight differences in the two person team. A solo canoe (C-1) also has a swept in bow and stern but is wide in the middle section where the paddler sits. Carbon fiber paddles are much lighter and more efficient than wooden ones. These composite paddles have a bent shaft design which allows you to keep the blade vertical in the water for a longer part of the stroke. This gives you more power with each stroke. Fast boats need fast paddles. Try one and you'll agree.

Unlike a standard canoe, the seats in racing canoes are adjustable and can be moved either forward or backward. This is important for "trimming" a canoe — making it lay flat in the water while moving — and will come in handy during pregnancy as you will see in a minute. As a canoe moves in the water, it tends to sink more in the stern (rear of the boat) so you adjust the seat(s) to account for this. The seats are padded for comfort and to prevent sliding. Women may want to put some extra padding where their ischial tuberosities (two bones you sit on) hit the seat. Foot braces provide added stability. Drinking systems consist of jugs and tubing for "no hands" drinking and are part of every racing canoe. Replenishing fluids is important for distance racing.

Rowing began as an intercollegiate sport for women in the sixties and seventies. It became an Olympic sport for women in 1976. Since then, women at all levels, high school, college, clubs, and masters participate in crew. Shells come in one, two, four, or eight persons models. Sculling is rowing with two oars per oarswoman. Sweep rowing is rowing with one oar per person on the right or left side of the shell. Events are classified as heavyweight (shells with a rower weighing more than 130 pounds) or lightweight (all rowers weight less than 130 pounds). The rower slides fore and aft on the seat with each stroke. When you place the oar in the water (catch phase), flex your knees, hips and back and extend your elbows. Your legs, as well as your arms, chest, and back help to power the shell during the propulsion phase when the oar(s) pulls you through the water. Watching a shell moving through the water makes you appreciate the rhythm and pulse of this water sport.

PADDLING OR ROWING DURING PREGNANCY

Whether you paddle or row competitively or recreationally, you can safely continue either of these activities by making some minor adjustments and modifications during your pregnancy. Now is the time to tame your adventurous spirit and stick with calm waters on a familiar lake or flat river. Avoid strong currents, fast water or heavy boat traffic. In windy conditions, it's best to stay closer to shore to lessen the effects. Always paddle or row with a partner. Carry a PFD (personal flotation device) or wear it if you are not a strong swimmer. Dress for comfort and ease of movement. A T-shirt over cycling shorts or shorts with an adjustable waist band works well. Protect yourself from the sun with sunblock, a hat and sunglasses. Water sport shoes or light running shoes are fine. For cooler weather dress in layers and wear light gloves. Always carry water on board.

Be prepared to make some adjustments. If you are in a racing canoe, either a C-1 or C-2, you will need to adjust the seats as your weight changes over the next nine months to keep the boat moving level. Getting in and out of one of these "squirrelly" canoes can be tricky at eight or nine months. Take it slowly. Your stroke will change due to the bulk of the baby, especially in the sitting position. You will not be able to rotate your torso as much and may need to shorten your stroke a bit. If you are in a two-person canoe, you will set the pace. Keep the strokes steady and easy. Avoid speedwork or sprints.

Rowing, also a non-weight bearing activity, is a great sport to continue during your pregnancy, either indoors on a rowing ergometer, or on the water in a shell. Rowing, unlike paddling, involves both upper and lower body movements. Sculling or sweeping involves flexion of your knees, back and elbows. Practice good technique and modify if necessary to avoid injury to your relaxed joints and ligaments. For instance, you'll need to shorten your stroke in later pregnancy due to the "second passenger." You may need to reduce the load of rowing by shortening your oars or increasing the inboard length or flex of the oars, although doing this may cause the oar to land closer to your abdomen. Rowing on an ergometer has the added advantage of keeping you cool from the

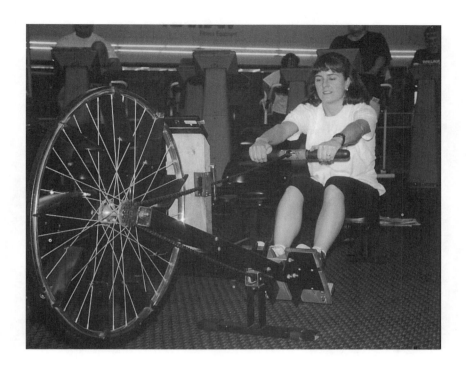

You'll need to shorten your stroke in later pregnancy due to the "second passenger."

backdraft of the flywheel. Put on a pair of headphones for entertainment. Keep a water bottle at your side and stay at a comfortable pace.

Susan, an experienced marathon canoe racer, paddled throughout her first pregnancy. In her first trimester she did shorter races at a comfortable pace and stayed well hydrated. For Susan, paddling felt very comfortable, more so than running where she experienced Braxton Hicks contractions in the last trimester. She attributes her triumph, Stella (eight pounds), delivered after a 21 hour labor, to her physical fitness and mental toughness. At last word, Susan is pregnant with her second child and coaching cross country running from the seat of her mountain bike.

Judy, a 41 year old mother of three and former Olympic rower, rowed throughout her pregnancies. She also continued to cycle,

run, and cross country ski. Judy reduced the intensity of her workouts and used a heart rate monitor during exercise for two of her
pregnancies. "I kept my peace of mind and was more concerned
with the baby's and my health than staying in tip-top condition."
Her labors were short, four to six hours. According to Judy, "Being an athlete helped me to deal with the discomfort better."

10

CYCLING

"It's like riding a bike, you never forget how." The saying is true — once you've learned how to ride a bike, you never forget. Think back to your early years on a bike — the thrill of peeling off on your own power down familiar roads and trails, the sense of control as you cut sharp corners and powered up hills. I still remember some of the rides I took on my bike as a young girl. The ride down the cemetery path that ran along side a stream always smelled like cedar. I remember what it felt like bouncing over cedar roots on my blue bike.

If you are like me, you'll recapture some of those moments every time you get on your bike. When you pause to take in a beautiful sunset or feel the thrill of flying down a hill pell-mell, you are reaffirming that you never forget how to ride a bike. Thousands of women today are enjoying the sport of cycling for the physical challenge and the sheer fun of riding.

Riding a bike is not only fun but it has its health benefits too. Since cycling is a non-weight bearing activity, it "spares" your joints and ligaments while providing many benefits. Your heart and lungs become more efficient at pumping oxygen to the working muscles in your legs. If you use pedal straps or a cleated shoe, your legs become stronger as they pull the pedals around each stroke. Your upper body is basically in a static position, nevertheless your back, arms, and abdomen are all working to hold you upright as your legs do the work of pedaling. Cycling, especially when combined with other activities like running, or swimming, is a great way to stay healthy and fit.

Cycling has mental benefits also. The women cyclists I spoke with convinced me that "runner's high" has its biological equivalent in cycling. The feelings of elation, contentment and confidence are common for dedicated cyclists. Cycling outdoors rewards you with the sights and sounds along your journey and a chance to clear your head. Whether you ride a mountain bike or road bike, you'll find freedom and adventure when riding.

Before we talk about cycling in pregnancy, I want to discuss cycling in general: types of bikes, proper fit, equipment and clothing, and safety issues. A discussion of these points will help you make a safe transition from cycling solo to cycling for two.

TYPES OF BIKES

As the interest in cycling has grown, so has the industry of bike designs. The bikes we learned on seem obsolete, replaced by a variety of models that fit each person's lifestyle and fitness goals.

Sport Touring Bike

Once the most popular type of bike (before the advent of mountain bikes), a sport bike still provides an economical entry into cycling. It usually has ten or twelve speeds and **is** suitable for either recreational or fitness riding. Novice racers may start with a sport bike and then move up to a racing bike.

Loaded Touring Bikes

If you have a travel bug, this is the bike that will get you there and back. These bikes are designed to carry panniers (large bike bags) or bike racks. Touring bikes have a longer wheel base (the distance between the center of the front axle and rear axle) which makes the ride smoother. A third chainring adds extra low gearing for climbing hills. You need this low gearing when you're riding with twenty or thirty pounds of gear.

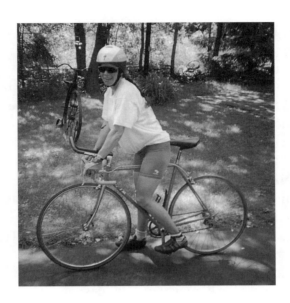

Returning from a ride on a racing bike.

Racing Bikes

Racers want to go fast, and these bikes are designed to do just that. The gearing is narrower, which means that it is geared higher for speed. The high pressure, narrow tires meet less resistance on the pavement. "Aero" bars are popular with triathletes and time trialists. They reduce wind resistance by keeping you riding low.

Mountain Bikes

These bikes have gained a lot of popularity — in fact, way over half the bikes sold these days are mountain bikes. Equipped with fat tires, upright handlebars and a triple chainring for wide range gearing, mountain bikes are designed for rugged terrain — whether it's climbing a rocky pass or descending a mountain trail. They also are great around town if you like to sit upright and ride on wide stable tires.

Hybrid Bikes

Hybrids are a cross between a mountain and road bike. Sturdy enough to handle more rugged terrain (fat tires, wide range gearing), they also can cruise along paved or dirt roads at a good pace.

CORRECT FIT

No matter what type of bike you're riding, correct fit is essential. If you're not comfortable, you're not having fun. Incorrect fit can lead to injury and frustration. The first bike I bought did not fit properly. The salesperson had me straddle the top tube to measure the clearance between the crotch and tube (one to two inches) — and that was it. I never felt comfortable on the bike. Before buying my next bike, I did some research.

Most bikes are designed around male anatomy. Our bodies have some significant differences which need to be considered when fitting a bike. We have shorter arms and torso, longer legs, narrower shoulders, a wider pelvis and smaller hands. How do you get a bike that fits correctly and handles well?

One option is a custom bike. If you're a competitive cyclist, you may already have a custom bike designed to fit your body. (Find a designer who is familiar with women's anatomy.) Another option is to "retrofit" a bike. A Fit Kit™ is a fitting aid which can help you do this by making adjustments to fit your proportions. A common practice for women is to replace the handlebar stem with a shorter one. This brings the handlebars closer to the seat to accommodate our shorter arms and torso. Check with your local bike shop. I used a Fit Kit™ when I bought my second bike. I bought a frame and then built the bike around my proportions.

What about a bike designed for women? Terry Precision road bikes have smaller front wheels (24 inches), paired with a standard (27 inch) rear wheel. The shorter top tube is more compatible with our smaller torsos. These bikes are popular with some women. Many manufacturers are now coming out with smaller-sized bikes.

Besides proper frame size, you need to consider a few other things to ensure a comfortable ride.

Saddles.

It's important to ride on a saddle that fits you and your riding style. Your pelvis is wider than a man's. The bones you sit on (ischial tuberosities) are further apart and may need a slightly wider seat. Many saddle manufacturers make "women's" models which are a little shorter and anywhere from a little to a lot wider than regular saddles. You can buy "anatomic" seats which are slightly wider and shorter and have extra padding for the ischial bones. Some of them have cut-outs or perforations in the saddle shell which, along with the shorter nose, help alleviate some of the pressure of the contact points. Terry Precision, a women-owned company, makes a line of saddles which are popular with many women riders. Check out the saddles and find one that is comfortable.

A common error novice riders make is to ride with the seat too low or too high. Remember, whenever you adjust the saddle height, you are altering the action of every muscle involved in pedaling. Set your seat height by sitting, without shoes, on the seat, placing the pedal at the bottom of the stroke. Your knee should be slightly bent. (It helps to have your partner or a bike shop technician do this with you.) Your saddle should be level to distribute your weight evenly.

Pedals.

Efficient pedaling requires that your feet be properly placed on the pedals. The strapless pedal binding system is a great improvement over the toe clip and allows you to fine tune the placement of your feet. You can prevent injuries, like knee pain, by fine tuning the angle of your cleats. A Fit Kit can help you properly align the cleats on the shoe. Toe clips require that you reach down and release the straps; to release from strapless pedals, you just rotate your heel outward. Many cycling shoes are compatible with the newer binding systems.

EQUIPMENT AND CLOTHING

Never ride without a helmet. Whether you have a mountain or road bike, you need to protect your head. Over 75% of cycling deaths result from head injuries. You're also setting an example for younger riders. Fortunately, most states have established laws that mandate helmets for children. Make sure your helmet is either ANSI or SNELL certified.

If you do much cycling, flat tires are inevitable. You're cruising along, enjoying the ride, and the next thing you know, you are sitting beside the road, fixing a flat tire. Always carry a spare tube, tire levers, and pump. CO_2 cartridges are handy for fast inflations. Practice a tire change at home beforehand.

Sun glasses protect you from ultraviolet rays but they also keep flying objects — like bugs — out of your eyes. The wrap around style usually works best. Again, glasses are usually designed for men so try to get a narrower frame that fits comfortably.

Drink before you go and carry water on your rides. Dehydration can be dangerous, especially in hot and humid conditions.

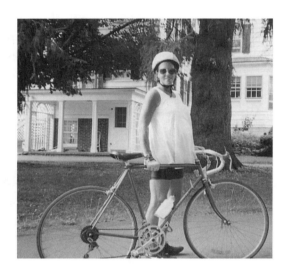

Ready to go with helmet, sunglasses, water, and comfortable clothing.

Cycling clothing is comfortable and aerodynamic. Non-restrictive lycra shorts and jerseys are the most popular. Buy shorts designed for women which avoid center seams and are usually lined with a cotton blend or fleece fabric. The back pockets on cycling jersey are handy for carrying quick snacks, identification or keys. Besides lycra, jerseys are available in a variety of fabrics with less "cling." Cotton T-shirts work fine with a supportive bra. Some women like the baggy shorts with a crotch lining for mountain biking or touring. Bright colors are a good safety feature.

In cooler weather, some of us head indoors (see Indoor Cycling) while the rest of us just add layers. You can wear a pair of lycra tights over your cycling shorts and then peel them off once you've warmed up. There are a variety of fabrics and designs for jackets and tights which wick away moisture to keep you warmer. Shoe covers keep your feet warm.

Cycling gloves prevent blister and "road rash" — the painful outcome when skin meets pavement. A gloved hand can also brush off debris from your tires. The fingerless style is great for warmer weather but you will want a full glove with a good grip in cooler temperatures.

SAFETY

Sharing the road is the credo of cycling. But remember, you're sharing it with big heavy objects! Stay alert and ride defensively. Here are some general safety tips.

- Obey all traffic rules. This sounds simple but there are times when it's tempting to blow through a stop light or signal. This attitude not only doesn't help relations with motorists — it is also dangerous.
- Stay to the right except in turn lanes when you want to give way to turning vehicles.
- Ride single file and stay as close to the shoulder as possible.
- Signal your intentions with hand signals.
- Watch for road hazards like potholes, rocks, gratings, and rail-road tracks. A triathlete friend had the misfortune of being thrown from her bike while crossing railroad tracks during a race. She suffered a fractured clavicle. Always approach tracks head on and not at an angle.
- Stay alert. Leave your headphones at home.
- Deal smartly with dogs. A blast with your water bottle or a verbal counter attack — (GET BACK!!) may ward off the bark-ing beast. Small blast horns are available that fit in the palm of your hand and send off a piercing "stop dead in your tracks" noise. You can always dismount and place your bike between you and the dog.
- Ride with a partner when possible. Avoid isolated roads or trails or riding in the dark.

- Always let someone know your cycling route. Carry identification and spare change.
- Keep your bike tuned up and ready for the road or trails.

TWO ON THE BIKE

Cycling during your pregnancy is a great way to stay in shape. As mentioned earlier, because it is a non-weight bearing activity, you reduce the risk of injury to your relaxed joints or ligaments. As your pregnancy progresses, your changing center of gravity and increasing weight may make cycling a better option than running or cross country skiing. Perhaps cycling is already a part of your fitness program or an activity you pursued while nursing a running injury. Whether you have a road or mountain bike, or even a tandem, you can continue to cycle with modifications and adjustments. Be sure to check with your health care provider about your cycling program.

Your fitness goals for cycling will change during pregnancy. You are now riding to maintain fitness, not to train for competition. This can be a difficult transition if you are a competitive cyclist. A few experienced cyclists I spoke with said that they "participated" in short citizen's races during the first few months of pregnancy. They cycled at a moderate pace (they were not racing) and stayed well hydrated. They were cycling for fun and fitness.

Kathy, a cyclist for fourteen years and competitor for the last six years, felt a mixture of feelings early in her pregnancy. She was thrilled to be pregnant but also felt jealous of her former training partners as they cruised by her on their bikes early in her pregnancy. It helped for her to realize that her condition was temporary and the health of her baby was far more important. She continued to ride during her pregnancy, stopped all "training" and enjoyed riding for pleasure and fitness.

CYCLING IN EARLY PREGNANCY

During the first few months, nausea and fatigue may cut your desire to exercise. Cycling may not sound appealing, but walking or swimming might be a good alternative. Some cyclists felt better getting outdoors in the fresh air. One competitive cyclist told me that she lost some of her ambition to ride in the early months due to fatigue. She rode less, cut back her mileage and felt better by the fourth month. Listen to your body in these first few months. Don't push it and be flexible.

Urinary frequency and breast tenderness are common symptoms during pregnancy. Empty your bladder before a ride and try to plan a route where you can get to a bathroom or "outdoor facility." You might want to wear a small mini-pad just in case. Don't cut back on fluid replacement. Your body needs this to prevent dehydration and overheating. You need to drink at least 16 ounces of water for every hour of cycling. Avoid the sports drinks. Replacement drinks contain ingredients that are not necessary for moderate levels of exercise and their use in pregnancy has not been studied. They also may upset your stomach. One competitive cyclist, who usually drank sports drinks while training, told me that she was unable to tolerate this during her early pregnancy. "It made me even more nauseated while riding," she said. On the same note, avoid cycling in very hot or humid conditions. A supportive bra or sports bra will help with tender breasts. A lycra top may feel too restrictive and uncomfortable so try a cotton T-shirt or loose fitting top.

Always stretch before getting on your bike (see Chapter 5). Focus on your hamstrings, calf muscles, Achilles tendons, hip flexors, neck and shoulders, and lower back. Start your ride spinning in easy gears. Likewise, at the end of the ride, shift to a cool down pace and replenish fluids. After long rides, be sure to eat some carbohydrates shortly after your cool down.

CYCLING IN LATER PREGNANCY

Your increasing weight and expanding abdomen, when coupled with your fetus's activity and position, may make cycling uncomfortable during the last few months of pregnancy. Many cyclists I interviewed had to alter their riding positions at this stage. Instead of riding on the drops (the lower portion of the drop handlebars), they rode in a more upright position with their hands on top of the handlebars. This gives more clearance for your abdomen, more room for lung expansion and puts less pressure on your hands. Some women switched to a mountain bike for the same reason.

When you ride on the drops, your hands and arms bear a good portion of your weight. Pressure on your hands, combined with the normal soft tissue swelling in pregnancy, can lead to nerve compression problems. The symptoms are numbness or tingling of the fingers, usually more painful at night. Let your health provider know if this is happening. Treatment is usually a wrist splint and ice packs.

Making some minor adjustments on your bike will make your ride more comfortable. Try moving your seat slightly forward to reduce the reach to the handlebars. Realize that by doing this, you are changing your pedaling form. Keep the adjustments small. If you normally ride with aero bars, you may need to replace them with a traditional handlebar set. Aero bars can be "squirrelly" — a little less stable. When I found out that I was pregnant, one of the first things I did was retire my aero bars.

If you suffer from hemorrhoids, sitting in the saddle can be uncomfortable. Try one of the anatomic seats or a wider seat with extra padding. Lower back ache is common in the last trimester. Strong abdominals as well as good posture and body mechanics will help prevent this problem. If back pain develops while riding, try different positions and maybe shorten your rides. Be sure to stretch your back before and after riding.

Braxton Hicks contractions, rhythmic tightenings of the lower abdomen, are common in the last trimester. Some cyclists experience these while riding, especially on longer rides. When these occur, slow down and focus on taking deeper breaths. If you're cycling on the drops, you are squeezing your diaphragm by both your position and your growing uterus. Your breathing becomes more shallow. Try riding in the upright position or get off your bike, take a short rest ,and drink some water.

Cycling may aggravate varicose veins. Because you are in a sitting position, you are further restricting blood flow to your legs. Support hose or lycra tights will provide some support. You will need to shorten your rides or switch to another exercise if they are severe or worsen with riding. Varicose veins in the vulvar area may be too uncomfortable for cycling altogether.

Vaginal yeast infections are common in pregnancy because of the rise in pregnancy hormones. Cycling can really irritate the situation because of the warm moist environment of cycling shorts and the friction of the bike seat. Change your shorts immediately after a ride. Try to wear shorts with the most "breathable" crotch lining. Select fabrics which wick away moisture and are comfortable. Consult with your health care provider if this becomes a persistent problem.

HOW FAST? HOW FAR? HOW LONG?

The answers to these question are individual. It will certainly depend on the health of your pregnancy and your level of fitness. Your cycling ability changes from early pregnancy to the last few months. Your added weight means that you have to work harder to cycle. When cycling for two, you need to listen to the messages your body is sending.

Certainly you will need to avoid any anaerobic workouts like sprinting or intense speedwork. It's safer to ride at a constant level of intensity. Keep your workout at about 60% to 75% of your maximal heart rate. (See Chapter 3.) That's a "somewhat hard" workout, between 12 and 14, on the Rate of Perceived Exertion scale. Do not cycle to the point of exhaustion. If you need to rest right after riding, then your workout was too intense.

The distance you ride will depend on again your level of fitness and other factors like terrain and weather. Avoid steep hills and rough terrain. Choose rides that have smooth road conditions and alternate route options, in case you want to shorten the ride. We don't know the effects of polluted air while exercising in pregnancy, but use common sense. Don't cycle during the worst periods. If it's hazy, hot, and humid, cycle early in the day or indoors on a wind trainer with air conditioning. Drink plenty of fluids.

I continued to cycle up to the day before I delivered — but with lots of modification. My pace slowed, and I tried to avoid steep hills and longer rides. My husband and I usually cycled together. We would agree on a route and then start out. He would cruise ahead and as soon as he was out of sight, circle back to me. I was glad we were able to both enjoy riding, and I know that he felt better knowing I wasn't cycling alone — which brings us back to the subject of safety.

All the safety issues previously discussed apply when cycling in pregnancy. Follow the rules of the road and carry identification and spare change. Avoid riding alone. Cycle with someone who matches your pace or do the "loop back" routine. Carry snacks and drink plenty of water. Stretch before and after your ride. Try to concentrate on good cycling form while making "comfort adjustments" as necessary. Be flexible. Listen to your body for any of the following warning signs:

- Shortness of breath, dizziness or chest pain.
- Signs of labor: Regular contractions or leaking of water from the vagina.
- Vaginal bleeding.
- Decreased fetal movement.
- Pain in the hips, back or pelvic area, or numbness around the perineum (vaginal area).

INDOOR CYCLING

If you live in a part of the country where you can't cycle year round, or if you feel safer off the road or trail, then indoor cycling is a good alternative. An indoor bike is available year round, and in the later months some of you may feel safer on a stationary bike. Changes in your sense of balance or poor weather can make indoor cycling sound appealing.

If you've never ridden a stationary bike, your first thought may be "BORING." Well, it can be, but find some interesting diversions like listening to music, reading, watching television, or letting your mind drift. Your thoughts may wander to your growing baby as you make mental lists of baby equipment. Also, video programs are available that simulate a bike ride.

A resistance trainer uses the back wheel of your bike to drive a resistance element. On a wind load simulator, the back tire makes contact with a shaft that turns a "squirrel" cage. A quieter model uses a magnetic device which rubs against the back tire. You can adjust for different levels of resistance. Place a board under the front wheel to keep your bike level and to avoid strain to your lower back. Rollers are a bit more tricky and probably not a good idea during pregnancy. You balance your bike while riding on top of rollers. A magnetic resistance unit is often attached to create resistance. A cloth shield will shield your bike from sweat. Always ride in a cool room with fans or air-conditioning.

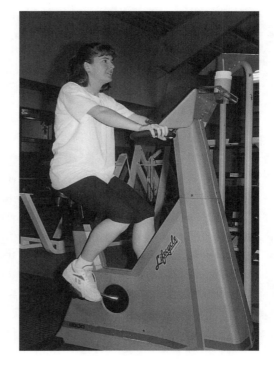

Try a computerized cyle
for some variety.

Health clubs generally have an array of computerized cycles. These can challenge your boredom with a variety of programs. While you monitor your performance, you can compete in a road race, ride on different types of terrain, or spin along at a steady pace. Fit is a problem with computerized cycles. The same "fit rules" apply as we discussed earlier. Check your seat height and the tilt of the saddle. Use the toe straps if available. You can adjust the handlebars in some models.

CLOTHING

Early in pregnancy you can wear your regular cycling attire. A supportive bra or sports bra will help alleviate tender breasts. In the heat you will want to wear breathable lightweight clothing. Cooler weather requires layering and fabric that wicks away moisture. In pregnancy you tend to perspire more. Keep that in mind when dressing for cycling.

Later in pregnancy, your expanding abdomen will probably still fit inside your cycling shorts if you go up a size. The traditional jersey may feel too restrictive, so try a large T-shirt that covers your abdomen. For safety, try to wear brightly colored clothes. Some women like wearing a maternity belt for a more snug feel to the abdomen. Don't forget sunglasses, sunscreen, and your helmet.

KATHY'S PROGRAM

"Cycling has taken a back burner for now," says Kathy, a 31 year old mother of Rebecca, an active one year old. Before Rebecca's birth, Kathy, an environmental scientist, competed in United States Cycling Federation (USCF) races.

As a serious racer, Kathy averaged 200 miles a week with speedwork and distance rides. During the off-season Kathy cross-country skied, swam, and did weight training for lower body strength. With the news of her pregnancy, Kathy was both excited and concerned about how her fitness level and body would be changing over the next nine months. Before she was certain she was pregnant, she was surprised by how she felt "less power" while riding with other cyclists. These early changes were followed by sleepiness and fatigue in the first trimester. She cut down her mileage, took easier rides, and stopped riding for competition. "I didn't mind altering my exercise — my baby was more important. However, at times I was envious of my friends who were still training for competition."

During the second and early into her third trimester she avoided hilly terrain and began to walk more. Occasionally while riding, she felt a pulling sensation in her abdominal muscles which she relieved by riding more upright. By the end of her third trimester Kathy replaced cycling with brisk walks. After a nineteen hour labor, Rebecca, weighing eight pounds, one ounce was born. "I was hoping my fitness would help, but labor was more intense than any pain I had experienced during competition. I think my fitness level did help with my recovery. I was back cycling four weeks after Rebecca's birth despite having lost quite a bit of blood at delivery."

Kathy sums it up like this: "Cycling while pregnant is fine provided you listen to your body and know when to back off. Don't be uncompromising when it comes to riding position -- riding on the drops with the added girth of a baby isn't easy. Be willing to make changes in your position on the bike. Being an athlete enhanced my awareness of my body during my pregnancy. The balance between exercise, nutrition, and rest became more important while I was pregnant."

CINDY'S PROGRAM

Cindy came from a strong background in cross- country running but later branched out into cycling, marathon canoe racing, and triathlons. At 31, she was initially shocked by the news of her first pregnancy. Her thoughts turned to how her active life would change and how she and her husband would adjust to parenthood. "I became fired up about exercising during both my pregnancies and decided I could safely stay fit and enjoy being pregnant."

Cindy continued to run, cycle, and lift free weights in the first trimester, but fatigue sometimes forced her — wisely — to substitute rest for exercise. She felt more energetic in the second trimester, so she continued to cycle but reduced her running mileage. "I altered my bike routes to include fewer hills and made sure I drank plenty of water. As an athlete it was difficult adjusting to my changing body contours. I didn't like the 'pear shape' of pregnancy. Prior to pregnancy, exercise always boosted my self-esteem so I knew that if I continued to exercise safely, I would get through this temporary period with a positive attitude."

By the third trimester, running became more uncomfortable so Cindy continued to cycle and lift light weights. Instead of riding on the drops, she rode more upright making breathing easier. "I took easier rides and coasted for short rest periods. I never over-exerted myself."

Both of Cindy's labors were induced and long. "I think exer-cising and being fit gave me the mental edge and stamina for both my labors." Ariel and Alec, both healthy, weighed in at seven pounds, ten ounces and nine pounds, respectively. Cindy advises women to get in shape before pregnancy and maintain a flexible fitness plan that can be modified along the way. When I last spoke to her, I learned that Cindy was towing her two children in a bike trailer on the hills around her home. She and her husband are now expecting their third child.

11

WINTER ACTIVITIES

There is a popular 50 kilometer (31 miles) ski race in Central New York, called the Tug Hill Tourathon, which attracts cross-country skiers of all levels from across the Northeast and Canada. This annual event takes place in one of the most beautiful and snow-laden regions in the state. Cold air moving across Lake Ontario creates "lake effect" snow — a snow-making machine which dumps tons of snow over the whole area.

The first year I skied the race, a lake effect snowstorm made the car drive to the race treacherous. However, this didn't stop over 300 enthusiastic and determined skiers from lining up at the start. By then, the snow was coming down in large clumps, and the race directors told us that any tracks set earlier on the course were just a distant memory. As the gun went off, we plowed ahead through the ankle-deep fluffy snow.

Fortunately, the snow had tapered off by the 15 km mark, and about then, I noticed a bobbing yellow sign up ahead hanging from the back of a skier. Approaching closer, I read the words, "BABY ON BOARD." As I moved over to pass, I noticed the protuberance at her waistline. "She must be in her seventh month," I thought.

The pregnant skier was moving along at a steady pace, rhythmically striding, looking comfortable, and obviously enjoying herself. Skiers around her offered words of encouragement and praise. Little did I know that the next time I skied the tourathon, I would be five months pregnant and skiing with <u>my</u> baby on board.

If you live in the snowbelt, the months from November to April can be a challenge. As we discussed in Chapter 8, the shorter days, icy conditions, and snowy roads can make running dangerous, especially during pregnancy. One alternative to running in slush, doing laps in the pool, or riding a wind trainer, is to strap on a pair of "skinny skis" and venture outdoors to cross country ski.

Cross country skiing is one of the best "total body" workouts. Unlike some other sports like running or cycling, skiing works both your upper and lower body — all your major muscle groups. It is a low impact sport with little risk of injury. Downhill skiing, on the other hand, probably should discontinued during your later months of pregnancy. Your changing sense of balance can put you at risk for injury.

There are two basic techniques in cross-country skiing. Classical skiing is the traditional method of skiing. Your arms and legs move in an exaggerated running motion as you glide across the snow in grooved tracks. Freestyle skiing, commonly called skating, is a technique of skating on skis where you transfer your weight from ski to ski as you glide on packed snow. Let's talk a bit about the technique and equipment in cross country skiing and then we'll discuss skiing in pregnancy.

NORDIC SKIING FOR THE NOVICE

If you have <u>never</u> cross country skied, now, during your pregnancy, is not the time to begin (you might, however, skip to the snowshoeing section further on). Wait until next season when you'll be looking for ways to get back in shape. But if you have cross country skied a few times or have done some downhill skiing, the early part of your pregnancy is a good time to gear up and go. The "how-to's" of the sport are relatively easy. If you can walk, you can run — if you can run, you can cross country ski! Here's how.

EQUIPMENT

Getting the hang of skiing is easy and enjoyable if you have the proper equipment.

Bindings

New binding systems have taken the place of the old "three pin" system. Most manufacturers produce a boot and binding system that is not interchangeable with other systems.

Boots

Select a boot that feels comfortable. You will want a low cut, light boots for classical skiing. Freestyle boots are higher and offer more support for skating. There are now combi-boots as well as skis which are designed for both striding and skating.

Skis

Proper ski length depends on your size, skiing ability, and type of skiing you want to do. As a rule, classical skis should reach your wrist when your arm is raised overhead while freestyle skis will be shorter. For classical skiing you need to decide whether you want waxless or waxable skis. "No-wax" skis are popular with recreational skiers — just step onto the ski and go. The downside is that you lose glide and speed. Waxable skis can be "fine-tuned" to the snow conditions by applying different types of wax. Wax under the boot area of the ski provides the grip on the snow allowing you the traction to "kick" or push off. You apply glide wax to the tips and tails of the skis for striding and to the entire ski for skating. A new generation of waxes has simplified both kick and glide waxing but waxable skis still take much more attention.

Poles

Base your pole length on your height and on the type of skiing you will be doing. Make sure that your poles are not too short. Most good poles have a "right" and "left." The pole generally comes up to your shoulders for striding and for skating the "mustache rule" applies. (The top of the pole reaches the point between your mouth and nose.) The longer length gives you more power throughout the glide.

Visit a shop that specializes in nordic skiing gear. Take an experienced ski friend with you when you're shopping for equipment and ask questions. Look for "ski package" bargains as well as sales at the start and the end of the season. You might consider renting equipment or borrowing a friend's set before buying cross country ski equipment.

TECHNIQUE

As I noted earlier, if you have not cross country skied before, wait until after your pregnancy to start. Here are some technique tips that you can use then, or before your pregnancy.

Diagonal Stride

The diagonal stride is the heart and soul of cross country skiing. (Well ,maybe the "heart," — skating on skis is probably the "soul"). Striding in set tracks is the easiest way to learn the fundamentals. To begin, start walking on your skis and let your arms swing naturally, keeping your poles slanted backward. Get a rhythm going. Once you feel comfortable walking on your skis, try jogging. Push off with one foot and drive the other leg forward. The key to striding is the glide. You want to transfer your weight onto the gliding ski completely and "ride the glide." Keep your knees slightly bent and centered over your ski as you put pressure on your heel and bring your other ski ahead. Keep your strides short at first.

Practice without your poles. This forces you to concentrate on transferring your weight completely and to avoid the common errors of straddling between two skis or using the poles as crutches. Exaggerate your arm swing as you move along. Diagonal striding is like running — your right arm comes forward with your left leg. Keep a relaxed grip on your poles and keep the pole tips pointed backward a bit. When your arm comes forward, set the pole tip in the snow and give a little push — this is when you "plant" the pole. Keep your arms slightly bent, plant the pole in the snow and push as you drive past it. One of the best ways to learn, or to improve, is to shadow an experienced strider and mimic his or her movements. Consider taking a few lessons to master the technique. Soon enough, you'll be out on the trail enjoying one of winter's popular pastimes.

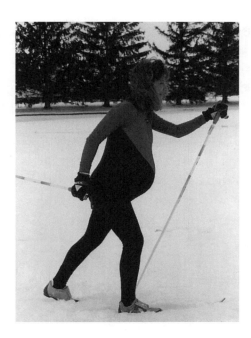

A good example of diagonal stride. The weight is over the
ski, the knee is bent, and the ski pole is planted in the snow.

What about skating?

Skating or "free technique" skiing is faster than classical skiing and lots of fun. We skate on open trails, like snowmobile trails,
where the packed snow provides a smooth gliding surface.
Groomed trails will often have a set of tracks running parallel to a
packed trail for skating. If you are an experienced nordic skier,
you are most likely familiar with this newer technique. Often called
skating on skis, it calls for you to transfer your weight from ski to
ski in rhythmic body shifts.

Proper weight transfer and balance are the keys to successful
skating. Beginners have trouble "committing" to the gliding ski
and instead straddle in between their skis, losing momentum. (It's
the same thing that happens in diagonal stride.) As you glide, try
to align your body (head, hip, and knees) right over the flat ski. A
flat ski is a fast ski. I try to keep my chin right over my gliding ski.

Just before starting the next glide, your recovery leg should move in close to your glide leg. At the same time, edge your gliding ski and push off. As the thrusting phase ends, your next gliding phase is beginning on the other leg. Practice by following a good skier, concentrating on shifting weight from ski to ski. Skating without poles can help you master the process.

Let's review some of the techniques used in skating. First is double poling. It is like the technique used in classical skiing where your skis are parallel and you push off with both ski poles at once. Double poling is used on slight downhills or as a change of pace.

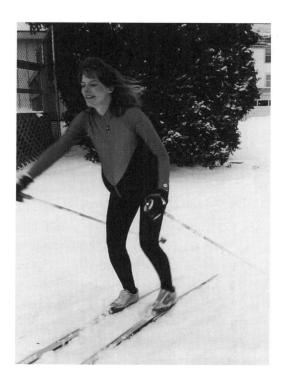

Double poling

V-1 skating is a double poling movement with every other skate. Generally, you pole on your stronger side and just skate on the other side. Diagonal V, similar to a herringbone where you alternate poling from side to side, is used on steeper uphills. There are other variations of skating technique — all aimed at skiing faster.

If you are an experienced skier, there is no reason for you to stop skating while you are pregnant — just watch your intensity level. If you are a novice, better stick with striding this season and give freestyle skiing a try next year.

For more information on equipment or technique, there are several excellent books and videos listed in the Resource section.

ONE PAIR OF SKIS — TWO SKIERS
Ski Touring

Touring is basically walking along at a moderate pace on skis. Except for steep hills or deep snow conditions, your rate of perceived exertion will probably stay in the "fairly light" (10 to 12 on RPE scale) zone. Ski with people who match your ability. Nothing is more frustrating than struggling to keep up with an energetic pacesetter — someone who has forgotten that the enjoyment is in the journey, not the miles covered. Set your own pace and take frequent water and rest breaks. Plan a tour that has options if you decide that you want to shorten the outing. A tour in the woods with your partner is a pleasant way to spend an afternoon, get some exercise, and enjoy the outdoors.

Diagonal stride

Classical skiing is safe for both the novice and advanced skier during pregnancy. As you know, your center of gravity and sense of balance has changed. You will need to make some minor adjustments to your technique, like shortening your stride a bit, in the later months. Some of you may find a waxless ski a better choice in pregnancy, giving you better grip but forfeiting a little speed. Obviously your pace will be slower and you will want to avoid steep or rugged terrain. Stay in the 12 to 14 zone on the RPE scale. You may experience mild Braxton Hicks contractions while skiing. Slow down or stop and rest.

Lisa, a competitive runner, cross country skier, and triathlete found that cross country skiing was a lot easier than running during her pregnancy. Her running pace slowed a bit but not so with skiing. She skied for the first fours months of her second pregnancy before the season ended.

Skating on Skis

If you are an experienced skier, you will probably enjoy skating on skis during pregnancy. As you might imagine, you will be aware of your added weight as you shift from ski to ski — much more so than in striding. Wendy, an accomplished skier and racer felt like she had "bad wax" while skating at six months pregnant. "It was difficult to move my body into good skating form," she said. "It seemed like a lot of work, especially on the uphills."

Shortening your glide and skiing on flatter surfaces will help. Skating is a more vigorous workout so avoid long steep uphills. You may need to switch to classical skiing in the last trimester if fatigue or lower abdominal pressure make it uncomfortable to skate.

Indoor Skiing

Indoor ski machines are another option when skiing conditions are poor or as a year-round workout option. Be sure to exercise in a cool room and drink plenty of water.

Ski Racing

A few cross country ski racers I spoke with raced in the first trimester. However, these women were all well-conditioned athletes, and they avoided overexertion. Gina, a competitive skier and mother of three, "went to the back of the pack and tried to ski in a relaxed and efficient manner." She reminded herself that she was a "participant" and not a "competitor" and avoided any prolonged aerobic stress, signaled by a breathless pace.

When I skied (not raced) the tourathon at five months, I kept a steady, relaxed pace. I drank plenty of fluids and snacked along the way. I was prepared to stop at anytime and paid close attention to my body signals. I remember feeling some mild back soreness near the end of the race which went away as soon as I got my skis off.

SNOWSHOEING

One manufacturer of snowshoes advertises: snowshoes are four-wheel drive for the feet. The new generation of aluminum and neoprene snowshoes are light and easy to use.

Snowshoeing is becoming more and more popular and can be

a good winter activity during pregnancy. You can enjoy the snowy landscape and don't need to have the skills of a skier. The "four-wheel drive" security is perfect when you have a changing center of gravity.

People often say about snowshoeing, as people did for cross country skiing, "If you can walk, you can snowshoe." It's true: no lessons are required to get out and snowshoe. There are a couple of technique tricks to keep in mind: When climbing a steep hill, push the front of the shoe into the snow first, engage the cleat, and push down. Make it like climbing a ladder. When descending, go heel first, setting the cleat to grip the snow.

Snowshoeing can be strenuous in deep snow and rugged terrain. Stay on easy trails and let your partner and others break trail. Drink plenty of fluids and plan rest stops.

There is no better way to experience the solitude of the winter countryside, and get a nice workout while doing so, than exploring on a modern pair of snowshoes. If you are not an experienced skier or skater, a set of brightly-colored hi-tech snowshoes may be the winter activity that fits you best during your pregnancy.

PREGNANCY TIPS FOR WINTER OUTINGS

Clear bright skies and sharp temperatures bring joy to the heart of those who like to get some exercise in winter. Don't be tempted to hibernate in the winter and wait for spring just because you are pregnant. Outdoor activity in fresh air is a good antidote for nausea and fatigue in the first trimester of your pregnancy. Even novices will enjoy the safe, low impact workout of cross country skiing or snowshoeing for at least part of pregnancy — unless you live where winter settles in for a full nine months!

Clothing

If you are a winter exerciser, you already know of the importance of proper dress. Cold temperatures and wind chill can lead to hypothermia (heat loss) and frostbite when you are exercising outdoors. It is even more important during pregnancy to dress appropriately and think ahead to conditions you might encounter.

Make sure that you dress in layers (How many times have you heard that?) Layers trap warm air and keep you warmer. For ski touring — which is much like a hike in the woods — and for snowshoeing, three layers works best. The first layer is thermal underwear -- the new polypropylenes are great "wickers" of moisture. A comfortable supportive bra is important. Lycra tights provide some added support to your lower abdomen, but you may like the feel of a prenatal abdominal support. These are available through mail order, or you can ask your health care provider.

Next, try a turtleneck or light fleece top followed by a wind resistant running suit. If you get too warm you can wrap the jacket around your waist. The elastic waist band on the pants should accommodate your abdomen. (You can always borrow a bigger size from your partner or friend.) For more strenuous skiing like striding or skating, you might want to wear lycra running tights (they stretch) over thermal underwear. Two pairs of socks, a light poly sock under a wool sock will keep your feet warm and dry. Hats and gloves are crucial — a bare head can throw off 25% of your body heat. You can take gloves off as you heat up and then put them back on as needed. I prefer mittens because of cold hands. Sometimes I use special hand covers which fit over the tops of the poles and create added insulation. Wear sunscreen and sunglasses if it's bright and sunny.

Dress for snowshoeing as you would for nordic skiing. — in layers. Wear a comfortable warm pair of boots and bring along a pair of ski poles. Wear windpants or a pair of gaiters to keep your legs dry.

Hydration

You may, because of the inconvenience of finding restrooms in the chilly outdoors, be tempted to skip a pre-exercise drink of water. Don't! Even though you may not be perspiring heavily, you still need replacement fluids. Every time you breathe you are losing fluids (respiration). You may notice this in very cold weather when your face mask, scarf, or hat is covered with frost and ice. Carry a fanny pack (or backpack if a fanny pack won't fit around your abdomen) with water and light snacks if you plan to be out for a while. Sip water along the trail. Wear a mini-pad if leaking urine is a problem.

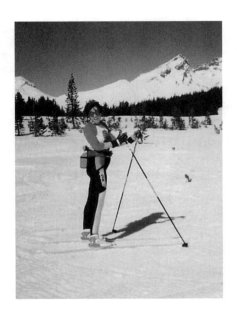

Carry water and food on every ski outing.

Where to ski

Since we rely on nature and not snowmakers for most nordic skiing, you obviously need to go where there's snow. Ski touring centers offer some advantages. The trails are usually groomed and graded according to difficulty. Restrooms and a place to warm up are available, as well as instruction. Golf courses, local parks, or snowmobile trails are other options. Be familiar with the area, bring along a map if possible, and never ski alone.

When to stop

Listen to your body to decide when it is time to switch to another activity or to reduce your outdoor winter activities. As one athlete said, "Let your body tell you how much is O.K. but know that some pregnancies require restrictions in activity."

Certainly, if you develop any medical complications (See Chapter 3), then you will need to restrict or eliminate skiing and snowshoeing. Keep your health care provider updated on your skiing activities and how you are feeling. If all is going well, you can continue a moderate level of these winter activities, while paying attention to hydration and rest, right up to delivery. Stop if you have pain, bleeding, leaking water, dizziness or other warning signs.

SANDY'S PROGRAM

Sandy, a mother of two teenage daughters, cross country skied as well as cycled and swam during both her pregnancies. Her first daughter was conceived while on a 2,500 mile bike trip through Europe and England. Despite some nausea and emotional ups and downs ("At one point I broke down crying when a truck came too close to me") she and her husband completed the trek without mishap. Sandy swam throughout her first pregnancy and then picked up recreational cross country skiing during her last trimester. She and her husband back country skied into state lands and parks. "On the very day that Amy was born, I had planned to ski with my husband and another couple. I had to call it off because I went into labor," Sandy said. The birth was uncomplicated and Amy arrived weighing seven pounds, one ounce.

It sounds hard to believe, but Sandy conceived the second time while on a bike trip in New England. (What is it with bikes?) This time she skied all winter during her second trimester and felt great. She said, "I don't recall having any problems. In fact I did a 5 mile citizens' race and felt fine. I never pushed it." Sandy's labor and delivery was rapid, about 5 hours, and uncomplicated. Katrina weighed eight pounds, four ounces. Sandy gained about twenty pounds with both pregnancies and was back to her pre-pregnancy weight by her six week check-up.

12

DELIVERY AND POSTPARTUM

SPECIAL DELIVERIES

Each woman's pregnancy and delivery will be different. There are many contributing factors, some of which are beyond our ability to influence. So it follows that the delivery experiences of active women are as varied as the women themselves. Being physically active and fit will not guarantee you a fast, painless, and problem-free delivery. The only consistent findings for women who exercised both before and during their pregnancies is that they tend to tolerate labor better. (Mittelmark et al. 1991, p.228)

Here are the labor experiences of some of the women I interviewed. See how they felt their fitness affected their delivery. (Baby's name and birth weight follows each quote.)

"I had good control and strength. I breathed through my labor (6 hours) the same way I did lifting weights." (Taryn, eight pounds, twelve ounces)

"Exercising regularly kept me focused during labor. I believe being in shape helped with the last stage. I had the energy to continue as labor progressed." (Samuel, eight pounds, three ounces)

"I was induced with Pitocin® because I was over-due. I had hard labor for four hours and then pushed for two hours. I think exercise gave me more endurance but may have made my pelvic muscles tight." (Justin, eight pounds, five ounces)

"I delivered Lindsey (my fourth baby) in my car three hours after my 3 mile. I had a nice and easy delivery! (Lindsey, nine pounds, ten ounces)

"My first labor was 19 hours. My second labor was 38 hours total — 12 were hard labor. I had expected an easy labor since I was "fit" but found it wasn't the case." (Daniel, eight pounds, nine ounces)

"I think being in shape made labor less strenuous and easier to handle. I had a VBAC." (Vaginal birth after Cesarean) (Conner, eight pounds, six ounces)

"Labor with my first was so intense. It began with pains a few minutes apart and continued through the night and morning. I pushed for about 3 hours before receiving a C-section. This takes an enormous amount of strength." (Travis, eight pounds, eight ounces)

"I could concentrate on the rhythm of my body without fear, especially when pushing for all my la-bors." (Sarah, seven pounds, two ounces; Forrest, seven pounds, two ounces; and Lillian, six pounds, ten ounces)

"My labor lasted 5 1/2 hours total. Two of those were hard labor. Delivery was so fast I wound up in the delivery room with no glasses and no camera." (Sean, eight pounds, thirteen ounces)

"I was tired during the labor because I had run that morning and climbed a mountain the day before, but I never had any real difficulty. Perhaps exercise taught me endurance and 'toughness.'" (Stella, eight pounds)

"I was fit so my recovery was very good. My first labor was the same length as one of our longer canoe races." (9 hours) (Vickie, eight pounds, nine ounces)

"I think exercise helped me through the pregnancy and was vital in my postpartum recovery. I don't think it helped me in labor other than I am very comfortable with my body and can isolate and relax specific muscle groups. Labor sure hurt more than any race I've run!" (Joseph, seven pounds, six ounces)

"I think being in shape gave me the stamina to go so long — 38 hours!" (Annika, six pounds, eight ounces

"I felt strong and had stamina and endurance during my 11 hour labor. I also had a positive attitude." (William, seven pounds, five ounces)

"Exercise definitely helped me get back in shape after Brianna was born. I started out weighing 112 pounds and ten days after the birth I was 112 again!" (Brianna, seven pounds, ten ounces)

Now that your nine month journey has ended with the welcome birth of your baby, you and your partner are beginning a new stage of labor — life with baby. If you kept fit during pregnancy, you are probably eager to "get it back" and resume an exercise program. Fortunately, for most fit women, it won't take another nine months to recover and get back your shape. But, before you get started, take a moment to reflect on the tremendous changes your body has gone through over the past nine months: the rigorous muscle stretching, the ligament and joint laxity, the increased blood volume and hormone surges, to name just a few. Now, your body is beginning the process of returning to its pre-pregnancy state. Let's first take a look at some of these postpartum physical and emotional changes, and then we'll talk about resuming an exercise program.

PHYSICAL CHANGES — PREGNANCY IN REVERSE

Your uterus, that amazing muscular bag, grew from three and a half ounces to nearly 2.2 pounds in weight. It will begin contracting, a process known as "involution," shortly after your baby's birth. These contractions, or "after pains," occur naturally and can be stimulated by breastfeeding. Your uterus returns to its normal size by about six weeks postpartum. Expect bleeding after birth lasting from two to four weeks. However, if your bleeding suddenly gets heavier, this may be a warning sign that you're doing too much and need to slow down.

Your pelvic floor muscles, the muscles that support your uterus, bladder, and rectum, were stretched while you were pregnant and during the delivery of your baby. If you had stitching for a large tear or episiotomy, expect the area to be sore for several days. You can sit in a warm shallow bath to get relief and to promote healing. Keep the area clean and dry. There's also a good chance that the leaking of urine may have been a problem near the end of your pregnancy and may continue now. Kegel exercises, which hopefully you practiced during pregnancy (by contracting the muscles around your vagina), will strengthen these important muscles and speed up the healing process of an episiotomy or repair.

Your abdomen — the focus of so much attention for the last nine months — is again the focus of your attention as you gaze at what probably looks like a loose bulge of flesh. You were hoping, I'm sure, that once the baby was out, you would regain a flat stomach again. It's going to take a little work for that to happen. I'll describe some exercises later in the chapter.

Your abdominal rectus muscles (the two up and down muscles) had the awesome task of stretching around your growing uterus. Diastasis recti, a separation of the muscles, can occur in some women and contributes to lower backache. It's important to begin abdominal exercises soon after delivery.

If you plan to nurse, get your baby on the breast as soon as possible. Your breasts will begin to leak colostrum, the pre-milk liquid that provides nourishment and antibodies. Your milk comes in by the third or fourth day postpartum. Frequent nursing and a good supportive bra will help relieve any engorgement. Wear a tight supportive bra and apply ice packs if you are not nursing and your breasts become engorged.

Lower back pain is one of the most common complaints in pregnancy and postpartum. It is important that you practice good posture and proper back care from day one.

Here are a few back care and posture tips:

- Stand tall — head pulled up, shoulders down. Tighten your buttocks and pull in your abdominal muscles.
- Wear a supportive bra.
- When sitting, press your lower back into the back of the chair. Try not to slouch.
- Place your baby on a pillow and rest your feet on a stool when you nurse. This raises the baby closer to you and prevents stooping over the baby. I set up a "nursing chair" with a pillow and small stool.
- Always think of your back when lifting or carrying your baby.
- Make sure stroller handles are long enough for your height (some models have adjustable handles).
- Front baby carriers should hold the baby snugly to your chest and have adjustable straps.
- Lift with bent knees, pull in your abdominal muscles, and tuck in your buttocks.

EMOTIONAL CHANGES — THIS TOO SHALL PASS

Giving birth to your baby requires that you go through your own rebirth in a sense. Once your baby leaves your womb, get ready to share what may be the strongest bond you will ever have with another human. That's not to say that this crossing over into parenthood is a non-traumatic step. Each step of the way will challenge you as you experience one of life's most important events. Prepare for these emotions and you may be more able to cope.

The first few days, weeks, and even months of your baby's life is a period of tremendous adjustment for the baby and for you. Even though you have been "expecting," suddenly, with no time to warm up, you seem to be in a new race — which can seem like a rat race. The adjustment to a new baby feels overwhelming to many active couples — especially if you are both used to a life of order and routine. As one swimmer and mother of six said, "It's not what babies do to your body — it's what they do to your life."

A new baby leaves no part of your life untouched. Your routines will be upset, schedules changed, and adjustments made. You may feel that you have no freedom and the responsibilities of parenting feel overwhelming. It's easy to lose your perspective among sleepless nights, a parade of visitors, and dirty laundry. You may feel blissful one minute and agitated or sad the next. What's happening?

THE BLUES

Like many new moms, you may begin to feel low two to three days after your baby is born. Your hormones (estrogen and progesterone) have suddenly dropped after the birth. Lack of sleep and an abundance of new stressors can lead to feeling down, depressed, or irritable. Now is the time to be easy on yourself and "take one day at a time." Look over the following suggestions for coping and give them a try. If you find yourself becoming increasingly depressed, don't hesitate to seek help. Talk to your health care provider or get in touch with "Depression After Delivery," a national support group. Write to P.O. Box 1282, Morrisville, PA 19067 or call (800) 944-4PPD.

COPING

Rest

The old saying, "rest when your baby naps" still applies. Accept any and all help from friends and family. I can remember how relaxing it felt to sit nursing my son as my mom buzzed around the house tidying up and doing laundry. From the very beginning, use the teamwork approach with your partner. Avoid the tendency to place "ownership" on the baby — doing everything yourself. Remember, it's a twenty- four hour job. Share the duties and be flexible. If you already have other children, make the most of catnaps or sitting down for a breather.

Support

Somehow six weeks has become the landmark for "getting back to normal." For the past nine months, you have practically lived at your practitioner's office, and now, suddenly, you're on your own. If you are returning to work outside the house, you'll add even more to the stress. Be sure to stay connected to family, friends, or other moms who know what you are feeling. Share your feelings with your partner and try to get some "couple time."

Nurturing — your baby and yourself

Caring for your baby is hard work. You need time out and time alone. Exercise is time well spent. It boosts your physical energy as well as refuels the mothering tank. If you are a list maker, stop now. Reviewing a list of undone things at the end of the day will just make you more frustrated. Instead, set some general goals and take advantage of those 15 minute snatches of time in between diapering, feeding, and bathing. I remember thinking how relaxing and restful my eight week maternity leave would be. I had visions of sitting in the yard, blissfully finishing a baby quilt I had started as my baby lay napping next to me. Guess what? The baby quilt is still not done two years later.

For Dads

You too are going through your own emotional passage. For nine months you watched and waited. Now, with your baby's arrival, you have the opportunity to learn about yourself as a father, partner, caregiver, and child-raiser. Right from the start, a hands-on approach is best. The more you do, the closer you will feel toward your child. Much of the early bonding to a baby comes with simply participating in the care and everyday (and night) routines. These early bonds are strong and provide the foundation for a healthy family.

Appreciate the tremendous physical and emotional changes your partner is going through. Patience is key. Give some leeway for the moodiness. Listen to her concerns and try to offer support. Maybe you need to put some of your needs on temporary hold. Give her the chance to go out for a run, walk, or paddle so she can return refreshed and feeling better about herself. This gives you the opportunity to spend time alone with your baby. The first few weeks are a period of incredible readjustment for both of you.

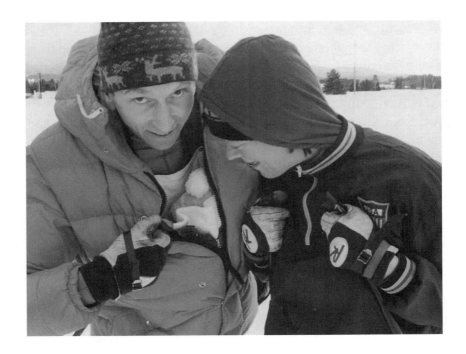

A new baby leaves no part of your life untouched.

EARLY EXERCISES

Whether your labor was long or short, vaginal or Cesarean, you can begin some simple exercises in the first few days. You are probably eager to jump back on your bike or go out for a jog. Hold on. Your muscles and connective tissue need time to regain strength and tone. Your joints and ligaments are vulnerable to injury, so you should avoid any jarring activities initially. For now, focus on your abdomen and pelvic floor muscles. Practice proper breathing techniques and stop if you feel any pain. Check with your health care provider before starting.

Easy abdominals

Lie on your back with knees bent, take a slow deep breath and, as you exhale, tighten your abdominal muscles. Try to hold the contraction for a count to five. Do ten repetitions a day.

Stay lying on your back with knees bent and feet flat. Press your back into the floor and slide your legs away from you while keeping your back pressed downward. Take a breath in, blow out, and slowly slide your feet back. Start slowly and build up to ten repetitions.

Pelvic floor exercises

Kegels

Your pelvic floor muscles need exercise even if you had a Cesarean. Concentrate on tightening the muscles around your vagina and hold for a count of 8 to 10. You can do this exercise anytime, anywhere. Work up to 25 repetitions during the day.

Pelvic tilt

This is a great exercise for good posture and relief from backache. Lie on your back with knees bent and exhale as you press your lower back into the floor and hold for a count to ten. Now inhale and relax. You can also do this standing while pressing the small of your back into the wall. Do ten repetitions a day.

LATER EXERCISES — GETTING IT BACK

Very little information currently exists about exercise during the postpartum period and during breastfeeding. One thing is certain, if you were active and fit during your pregnancy, you should be able to resume a gradual program before your six week checkup. Most physically active women do. But just like during pregnancy, you need to individualize your exercise program and discuss it with your health care provider. Your postpartum fitness goals are to heal, stay healthy, and start back gradually.

If you had an uncomplicated vaginal birth, you can probably start an easy program at about two weeks postpartum. Be aware of joint and ligament laxity which can last several weeks — sometimes up to three months. You'll be more pressed than ever for time but always warm up beforehand, even though it is tempting to skip the warm up and head out the door for your run. Try doing some stretches as you change into your exercise gear or as you are giving last minute instructions to the sitter. Warming up, cooling down, and stretching are integral parts of your workout so allow some time. Drink plenty of liquids, especially if you are nursing. Avoid exercises like cycling or paddling if you had an episiotomy.

Wait until you are pain free. Monitor your vaginal bleeding. If it suddenly gets heavier or starts up again, you need to back off and do less. So what <u>can</u> you do?

Whether you had a vaginal or Cesarean birth, you can begin walking right away. Gradually build up the intensity and duration. Enjoy the pleasure of walking with your baby and the opportunity to spend some time with your partner without distractions. At about two to six weeks, if all is going well, you might want to begin low impact aerobics or a special postpartum exercise class. If you had a Cesarean birth, then you need to avoid strenuous abdominal exercises until the inner layer of the incision has healed, usually in 4 to 6 weeks. Following surgery, it's not uncommon to feel some twinges and pulling sensations while exercising. Stop if you feel sharp pain. Wear a pad if leaking urine is a problem and remember: Kegels — Kegels — Kegels!

Low intensity stair climbing is another option as well as riding a stationary bike, treadmill walking, cross country skiing, paddling or rowing. All of these activities are low impact and you can easily modify them to suit your mood or energy level. Again, be very cautious of your vulnerable joints and ligaments and keep it light to moderate. What about swimming? Although swimming is non-impact you should wait to get in the pool until your bleeding has stopped since you will be wearing pads and not tampons. Your Cesarean incision should be entirely healed before resuming swimming so consult your medical provider.

Later, you can gradually integrate more jarring activities like high impact aerobics and running into your program. You can start walking and doing toning exercises with light weights and then work up to jogging or aerobics. Delay serious weight training until about six weeks after the baby. Elite and competitive runners I spoke with gradually started back with light jogging after vaginal deliveries in one to 4 weeks. Many breastfeeding runners commented on the challenge of running with larger or tender breasts.

Breastfeeding and exercise are very compatible. There is no evidence that exercise will diminish the quality of your milk, <u>and</u> nursing is a real time saver — no bottles or formula to worry about. Plan to nurse your baby right before you exercise, or if it's not time for a feeding, pump your breasts. Get a "megasupport" bra or try wearing two bras. "I went from an A/B cup to an E cup," reported one Olympic runner. Another elite runner would stop to nurse her daughter in the baby jogger while out for longer runs. Use nursing pads if leaking breasts are a problem. I cut up panty liners and stuck them on the inside of my bras. Some nursing moms told me that they felt more tired during the time they were breastfeeding.

Remember the importance of a balanced diet. Depending on your activity level, you need an additional 400 to 500 calories a day and lots of fluids (Cunningham et al. 1993, p. 256) -- 10 to 12 glasses. You may hear that exercise will cause your milk to sour due to lactic acid buildup. I wouldn't worry — if you exercise at a moderate level it is unlikely that this will happen. Besides, if you nurse before exercise you will avoid any such possibility.

Fit women like yourself are anxious to "get it back" — the fitness — but are just as anxious to "get it off" — the weight. After delivery, you will lose the weight of the baby, the placenta, and fluids, but you still will be heavier than you were before you became pregnant. But, since you are coping with so many things already, don't be concerned about weight loss for now. If you are not nursing, you can begin a sensible weight loss program. However, skimping calories is not wise, especially during the first six weeks when you need energy and stamina. A program of exercise and breastfeeding is no guarantee for weight loss in itself. Most active nursing mothers gradually lose the weight without really trying. But, it's not uncommon to carry a few extra pounds until you wean the baby. Follow a well-balanced diet (See Chapter 4) and be sure to get enough calcium, about 1200 mg. a day, according to RDA guidelines.

Whether you breast feed or not, take your time and be sensible as you move toward your prepregnancy weight. If you are not nursing, you may have started birth control pills for contraception. Some women claim that it is harder to lose weight while taking birth control pills. This has not been scientifically proven, especially with the newer low dose pills. DeproProvera,™ a progesterone hormone injection given every three months, is another form of contraception. This hormone may make it difficult to shed the last few pounds. Regardless of whether you nurse or bottle feed, or take hormonal methods of contraception or not, try to create a healthy balance of diet, exercise, and rest.

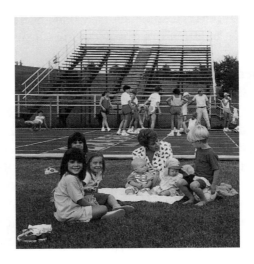

Babies and kids relax while moms get ready to run.

COMPETITION ... WHEN TO START

I read an article in a running magazine which suggested wearing a weighted vest during training. The theory was that the added weight increases leg-muscle power and speed without doing any special workouts. I couldn't help but think of pregnancy as a built-in "training vest." Does pregnancy make you a better athlete?

There are no studies to confirm if the physiological changes in pregnancy enhance athletic performance. Psychologically, there may be a positive effect. Track stars like Ingrid Kristiansen, Valerie Brisco, and Tatyana Kazankina all took their performance to new levels following their pregnancies. Valerie Brisco won two gold medals in the 1984 Olympics two years after having her son. Two years after her daughter's birth, Susan Notorangelo won the women's RAAM (Race Across AMerica) race.

Many competitive athletes have said that pregnancy, particularly labor, enhanced their mental and emotional stamina. For example, five months after delivery, Ingrid Kristiansen ran her fastest marathon — which she then improved upon the next year. She credits her family interests with helping her become a better runner. Other athletes agree. When you're a mother, you tend to use your training time more efficiently. You become more focused.

If you are an elite or professional athlete, you likely had special supervision of your pregnancy by your health provider. You probably, with luck, were able to plan your pregnancy during an off season. Most of the elite athletes I spoke with had just finished a vigorous racing season and were planning to get pregnant. One professional runner decided to get pregnant due to a broken foot. A competitive canoe racer went all out in the season previous to trying to get pregnant and placed second in the National Championships. "I wanted to do well because I didn't know when my next chance to race would be." Another marathon canoe racer conveniently had both her babies in December. She nursed and recovered during January through April and then started racing again in May. If you're like most active women I spoke with, you fit your athletic pursuits in around your pregnancy and the birth of your child — not the other way around.

Your return to competition is individual and dependent on your delivery experience and recovery. Regaining your prepregnancy fitness level takes time, and for some women, may never happen. Some competitive runners took one to two years to get it back. One 35 year old Olympic runner began racing after seven months but was plagued by fatigue and frequent viral infections. She realized that she was doing too much, too soon. She backed off and waited several months before racing again. After 21 months she clocked a 20:40 for a 4 mile race and later a 33:06 in a competitive 10K race. A former Olympic rower and mother of three returned to competition at three months and set a personal indoor record ten months later. She felt that her pregnancies did not provide a training effect, but being a mother brings a "focus" to her training. The time she does have to train is more intense and higher quality.

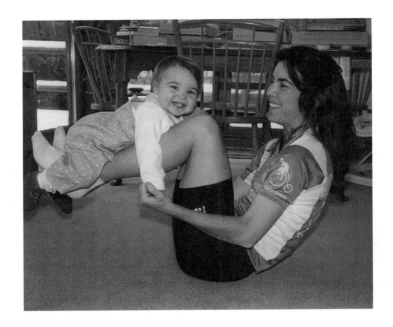

Getting back to your pre-pregnancy shape and
stamina is important but also very individual.

Whether you are a national-class athlete or an "around-the-block" jogger, you'll find that getting back to your pre-pregnancy shape and stamina is important but also very individual. Don't compare yourself to others or expect a miraculous comeback. The key to successful recovery is moderation, going slowly, and listening to your body. Remember, your body signals guided you through your pregnancy, and they will help you safely recover and get fit.

13

LIFE AFTER BABY — THE FIT FAMILY

Parenthood, as you are learning, is an on-going, ever-changing enterprise. Each day has new surprises, joys, obstacles, and challenges. You and your partner are discovering the realities of family life. No book or class can prepare you for life with your baby. In little time, you won't remember what life was like without your baby.

For many of you, returning to work is the next phase of adjustment. Safe, reliable child care is the cornerstone to the functioning of working families. Whether in your home, private home, or day care center, the best child care is what suits your family's needs. If your child is in a safe and happy care setting, you and your partner can start to develop strategies for fitting in exercise. But how?

Parenting is an elemental lesson in time management. You feel as if you have more and more to do and less and less time to do it. The key to survival is setting priorities and keeping your expectations in line. (Aim for the gold but settle for silver.) Now is the time for you and your partner to honestly discuss your fitness goals. Do you want to exercise for general fitness, weight loss, or competition? How many hours (or minutes) per day are "yours?" What options do you have to fit in 30 minutes — an hour a day? Do you prefer to exercise alone, with a buddy or in a class? If your partner is also active, how do your goals mesh?

FITTING IT ALL IN

Whether you are at home with your child (children) or working outside, finding time to exercise is a challenge. Perhaps you are home with two or three young children or your job requires travel or long hours, or both you and your partner are competitive athletes. Finding time to exercise while balancing family and work is not easy, but many active families are doing it. Here are some comments from a few:

"I am able to maintain a fairly good balance between family, work, and exercise because I am not driven to be the best at everything. I'm willing to sacrifice some things, like a perfectly clean house, for a chance to take Rebecca for a walk or go for a bike ride." (A cyclist.)

"Having kids has greatly reduced my opportunities for consistent exercise. Now that I am out of the habit of regular exercise, it is hard to get as motivated as I once was. My priorities are my family and home. Work is necessary, and exercise, while important, is difficult to fit in." (A marathon canoe racer.)

"With age and family I've gotten wiser about my training. I made a choice to stay home with my two children because I want to spend time with my family. A stationary bike, rowing machine, baby jogger, and pulk for skiing, as well as a cooperative husband all help me stay fit." (A cross country skier, triathlete.)

"Competition no longer seems like a priority as it once was. However, overall fitness is. I look at exercise as general body maintenance, like daily personal hygiene." (A runner, triathlete, marathon canoe racer.)

"I've learned that you don't need to do 'mega' miles in running to stay in shape. More miles is not necessarily better." (A triathlete)

"My priorities are very clear in my mind. My career has always been very important but I don't believe it requires 60-80 hours a week, and it doesn't make me as happy as my son does. Also, I manage stress at work much better when I'm exercising regularly." (A swimmer.)

"I continued to train and race throughout my wife's pregnancy; however, I think the intensity of my training decreased because I lacked her as a training partner. The racing and training became lower in significance. After our daughter was born, we were fortunate to have good friends who would baby-sit during periods that we wanted to train. When my wife got back into competition, my motivation and training improved." (A marathon canoe racer and cross country skier.)

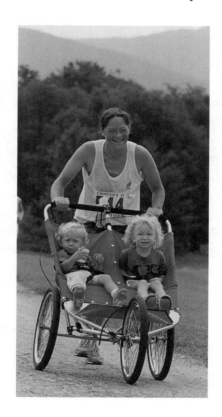

Some women are fired up to compete following their pregnancies.

GOALS

What are your fitness goals now that the baby is here? Many women I spoke with found that their competitive drive was diminished after having children. Training for competition requires a substantial time and mental commitment. It's natural that your priorities will change. Being fit and feeling good about yourself are important but may pale in comparison to the importance of your role as a parent. Parenthood may be a stimulus to move away from competition and continue your sport for fun — or an opportunity to take up a new sport(s).

On the other hand, some women are fired up to get back into competition following their pregnancies. Returning to competition gives you goals for your training program. An Olympic runner noted, "I have a supportive husband, a wonderful baby sitter, and a strong desire to race again at the same or higher level!"

Most of us will have a new perspective on exercise after having a child. Here, a former downhill ski racer and triathlete explains how her exercise goals have changed with parenthood.

My three-year-old points to the front of my T-shirt and asks, "What's that, Mommy?"

"That's a narwhal. This shirt was for Mom's swim team in Alaska, back when I used to get exercise."

I catch myself. Here I am walking down a trail in the woods, with the legs of my 30 plus pound son wrapped around my waist and my hands around his back, holding him in this conversational position. In my backpack, my twenty-pound one-year-old is jumping and leaning, trying to reach her brother's face and using my hair for extra balance. We've been walking this way for ten minutes and have at least five more to go. And I feel like I don't get any exercise?

It's funny, I reflect, how we reach our definition of exercise. My "formal training" started when I was eleven when I mowed a one-eighth-mile somewhat oval track in the field in front of our house. Every morning before school I would pop out of bed, don my "run-faster" Keds sneakers and head for the track. The routine set the approach I was to use for the next twenty-five years.

From age ten through college I was a competitive downhill skier. Cross-training was part of my personality so I varied my training daily and seasonally. I played field hockey and soccer, ran, lifted weights, went backpacking and biking, and engaged in many other sports. Nearly all my choices involved movement of my entire body and at least twenty minutes of sweat-producing, heavy-breathing exertion — that's what I call exercise.

After a setback from knee surgery, I became involved in competitive triathlons at age thirty. By this time, cross country skiing had become a passion, and I spent the long Alaskan winters with about two hours each weekday on the tracks and weekends telemarking in the backcountry. I balanced that out with long pool workouts, speed hikes of one to two hours with big elevation gains, ocean kayaking, biking, and a non-stop lifestyle.

By age thirty-six, I was back in rural New York, married, and still exercising formally and informally every day. My son was born in September after an active pregnancy of thirty-mile bike rides, firewood cutting and splitting, one-hour lap swims, and a long summer of active farming.

Then the priorities changed. There were still cross country ski outings that winter, but they were slower and shorter with the baby along. Summer bike rides now included scenic stops along the way and a mid-point picnic or exploration. Exercise for its own sake was replaced by easy-going outings with the baby. Quick naps, catching up on the bills, or making those necessary phone calls where I did not want to be distracted by kid noise or tugging, robbed me of those moments where it seemed I would be able to workout on my own.

My lifetime of being in shape carried me along. My upper body and back stayed strong from kid hauling. Our outings were frequent enough to keep my aerobic capacity up. In my few kid-free jaunts with non-parent friends, I was still able to keep up or even surprise them with my physical condition.

Now, with two children, the slow shift from what I still call "exercise" continues. Yet I feel going slower and answering the hundreds of three-year-old questions is more important. At home, I continuously scramble to stay on top of the basic life maintenance activities like food, dishes, bills, and laundry. My bike wind trainer and yes, even my skis gather dust.

This bothers me — a lot. But it is my choice. With parenthood, priorities have to be made and I did it this way. In my calmer moments, I consider these years just a different form of training. I am keeping, and even developing some strong muscles masses. Sleep deprivation and midnight wakings develop discipline to do things I really don't want to do, and the ability to perform even when dead tired. My endurance is probably better than in my triathlon days, because now my kid triathlons are often twelve hours long.

Probably the most important learning of parenting is that whatever you do, if you do it with some thought and conviction, then it is the right thing to do. Someday, I'm sure, I will be able to bike, hike, run, and swim hard again — maybe even competitively. Aerobic exercise will again be my norm. Or will it? I guess I don't dare predict. Whatever happens, it will be right.

Take some time to settle in on your fitness goals as you deal with the new demands on your time. Whether you choose competition or fitness, set some goals that will help you stay challenged and motivated while having fun.

FINDING THE TIME

Judy, a former Olympic rower and mother of three, shared with me her thoughts on setting fitness and family goals and finding the time for both. Here is her story:

At a women's gathering a few months ago, I listened to several mothers talk about making time to do something for themselves — like reading books, going out with friends, taking a course. "How do they ever make time for that?" I wondered. I marveled at their self-discipline and organization and couldn't remember reading anything other than books about kids in the last four years. I resolved to try harder to make that time.

But in the next few days, I realized that I, too, was taking time for myself — it's just that my priorities were different than theirs were. What I make time for is my exercise. My life has become busier and more intertwined with family, work, home, and community, yet I have clung to my workouts. They are my stress-relief, my head-clearing time, my health, my pleasure. Sometimes they are a time to be with friends, sometimes with my husband, sometimes alone, and sometimes in competition. There is a greater exhilaration and sense of strength that I get only from competition, and the goal of a race gives added incentive to keep quality in my workouts.

Sometime in the future I will again find time to read books and return to other hobbies — but even then, it won't be at the expense of exercise. It will happen when the demands of family and work have lessened.

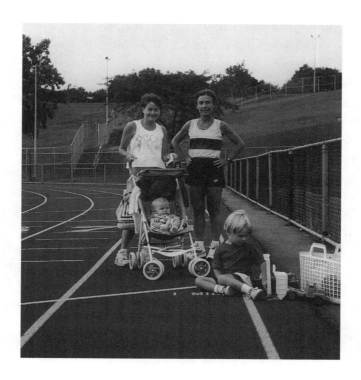

Maintaining fitness in an active family requires a substantial amount of teamwork.

TEAMWORK

Maintaining fitness in an active family requires a substantial amount of teamwork. Every family I spoke with stressed this point. There will be days when you will feel like anarchy has set in and defeat is just around the corner. Keep your perspective, for as they say, there is always tomorrow. You and your partner need to design your own strategies for meeting your baby's needs, doing household chores, and attending to the myriad of details that penetrate your daily lives. Mornings can feel like a strategic planning session as you discuss the day's plans and activities. Hopefully, part of that discussion is when, where, and for how long you will exercise.

A big change for some couples is spending less time training together. "I miss running with my husband. Now, we each take turns and occasionally run together if we arrange child care," says a mother of two. The teamwork concept will work if you are both able to share your expectations, and you are able to talk about those expectations. Think ahead, plan ahead and talk about it.

FLEXIBILITY

Flexibility — parenting gives new meaning to the word. It seems as if plans are always being changed by things like a sick child or a canceled sitter. Try to stay flexible. Look at these "crises" as an adventure in creativity.

Let's look at an example. You planned to run with the running stroller when your baby awakens from her nap. Now it's pouring rain. What are some alternatives? Why not hop on the wind trainer, start up an exercise video, or crank up the cross country ski machine? Use your athletic traits, determination, and fortitude to adapt to the new situations that are constantly arising. As one mother said, "Parenting is a form of cross training."

How flexible are you — not your joints, but your attitude? An area of debate is whether exercise is a positive or negative addiction. For some of us, the compulsion to exercise can become a negative aspect of staying fit. Missing a workout or having to change plans can bring feelings of guilt or disappointment. Obsessive feelings about exercise can erode the positive benefits such as stress reduction and a sense of well being. Some of the signs of addiction to exercise are: recurrent overuse injuries, weight loss, resistance to "cutting back," exercising through pain, and neglecting the other areas of your life. Only you know if you are losing the benefits by being too inflexible — by letting exercise assume too much priority, adding more stress to your life and your family.

Patty, a teacher and mother of two, has managed to squeeze exercise into her busy schedule:

Luckily I was able to take time off my teaching job after I had each of my children, so during their infancies I would organize the mornings so that I could run before my husband left for work. When I look back on those days, I remember firmly believing that mornings were the only time I could exercise, but as soon as I returned to teaching I realized I could not be rigid about exercising. I have to be at school by 7:30 A.M. and it is too dark and hazardous to run in the early morning hours, so I have learned to become an afternoon runner. Before my children were in elementary school, I would delay picking them up at day care so I could run or I would run just before dinner within the confines of our village. Now that my pre-teenage children participate in various sports and activities, I think my schedule - and theirs - is even more demanding so I used my "flexible maxim" to find time to exercise. For instance, when I take my daughter to flute lessons I always wear my running clothes and shoes. As soon as she enters her teacher's house, I take off and manage to run for thirty to forty minutes. I follow this same procedure when I take my son to tennis and lacrosse practice. Exercise after children is possible, but it can only be accomplished by being flexible and creative.

EQUIPMENT FOR THE FIT FAMILY

Many active families, using teamwork and flexibility, are able to pursue their fitness and even their competitive goals. Fortunately there is equipment available that will help you take your baby along while exercising. If you're thinking of buying any of these items, talk to someone who owns one and get their feedback.

Also, whether it's hiking, cycling, running or skiing, you'll need to do some extra planning for an outing with your baby. Remember the Scout motto, "Be prepared". Anticipate the need to nurse or offer a bottle, and carry spare diapers. Dress your baby warmer than yourself — you're moving and generating heat while your baby is still. Check the weather forecast. Use sunblock and hats with a visor for sunny weather. Grab a few toys for entertainment.

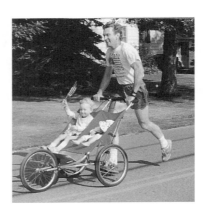

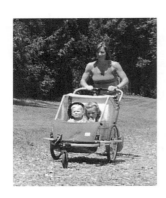

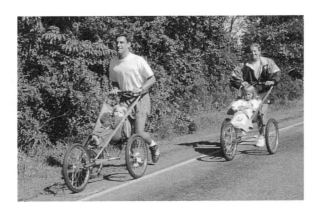

Running strollers in action.

Running strollers

There are different styles and models to choose from, and some even fold up for transport. Make sure yours has a braking system (handy when loading and unloading your baby), sturdy tires, and a leash in case your baby starts to get away from you. Some designs feature an infant bed. Canopies are handy, and you can also fasten a light towel with clothespins over the front to block sun or wind. It takes some practice running with a stroller. Your stride will shorten and hills can be a real chore. Try to keep a light touch and push with one hand so your other hand can still pump. There are double joggers for twins or your second child. One elite runner told me that she did hill repeats with her two year old and infant in a running stroller. Now that's a workout! Another Mom, who is an equestrian, not having a running stroller, pulled her children in a driving carriage for exercise. Her neighbors gave her some odd stares, but the children loved it.

Carriers

Front carriers are for infants, but once your baby can hold his/her head up, usually at three to four months, you're ready for a back carrier. Try one on with your baby before you buy. Make sure that both the shoulder and waist straps are comfortable. Carriers are great for walking, hiking, a stationary indoor bike, indoor rowing machine, and cross country skiing. We used our back pack for skiing with our son in good weather up until the age of two. Snuggled in the pack, he would usually fall asleep for a nap within the first twenty minutes of the ski. Having this kind of weight on your back requires strength and coordination and should be reserved for shorter outings on relatively flat terrain.

Bike trailers and child seats

Whether riding in a trailer or a child seat, your infant or child must wear a helmet. In some states it's the law — in all states it's common sense. You can put an infant care seat inside the trailer for added neck support. Some trailers also convert to strollers, though a little awkward, and can seat two children (maximum weight 80 to 85 pounds). They come in bright colors and you can place a safety flag on a long pole on the back. You'll find that you can pull bike trailers more easily with a mountain bike. Because a trailer is wider than your bike, avoid congested streets. There are retractable canopies and room in the trailer for snacks and toys.

Child seats are for one year-olds and up. A rear-mounted seat is safer than a front-mount and should have a seat back that isn't so high that it forces your child's head forward. Foot buckets keep toes away from spokes. When mounted, the seat should carry the child's center of gravity ahead of your rear axle. Go to a bike shop if you're not sure about proper mounting. A touring or mountain bike is more stable for carrying a child's seat. Before you launch with your precious cargo, try pulling an empty trailer or riding with a bag of potatoes in the seat. Get used to the added weight and negotiating turns and stopping.

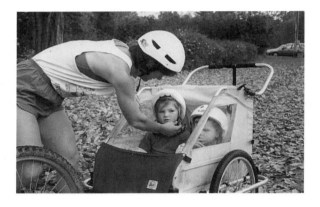

Checking helmets before starting out with a bike trailer.

Pulk

A pulk is a ski sled that you can pull while cross country skiing. The sled has runners which glide on groomed ski tracks and is pulled by a harness with a waist belt. A plastic shield protects your child from flying snow and wind. There's plenty of room to pack snacks and extra clothing in the pulk. Remember to bundle up your child and plan outings with "bail out" options if there is a change in weather or mood.

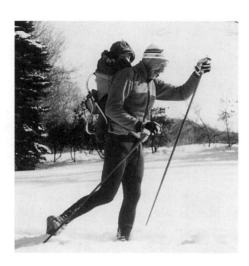

Two winter transport options
are a back carrier(left) or a
pulk (below).

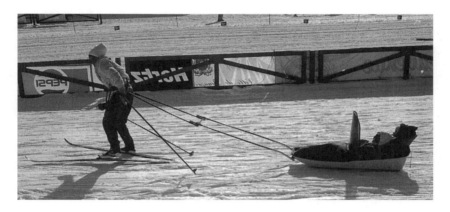

Machines and workout equipment

Weight stations, treadmills, steppers, cross country ski machines, rowing machines, stationary bikes, and climbers are all fitness options. Before you buy any piece of equipment , definitely try it out. Get a temporary health club pass and try their equipment to help you decide what you will enjoy and consistently use at home. Look for bargains in the want ads — there is a lot of "slightly used" exercise equipment gathering dust in people's basements. Get a flexible belt so that you can wear a cassette player. Music will jazz up workouts on any machine.

Home Fitness Equipment

A home fitness "center" can be as simple as an aerobics tape and hand and ankle weights or as sophisticated as a complete workout room with various workout stations and equipment. It depends on your budget and space limitations. Exercising in your home is backup for inclement weather or for a parent at home without child care arrangements. Getting some exercise in your home is a time saver, and as one mother said, "Something is better than nothing."

Videotapes

There is no lack of variety here — everything from stretching and toning to high intensity aerobics is available. There are also videos that will simulate a cross country ski, bike ride, or jog as you work out on your machine and visually escape to scenic areas like Switzerland or Hawaii (See resource section).

Fitness Centers

The growth of fitness centers is a reflection of the need for time-efficient and versatile exercise options for busy people. Most centers provide one stop shopping for instruction, exercise classes, state of the art equipment, and often, child care. Do your homework before becoming a member. Talk with current members, get a trial pass, and stop by at the time you will most likely use the facility. Are instructors certified? What is the child care like? Talk with other moms. How often will you go? Is it worth the investment? YMCA's or community centers are other options.

Finding Time For Fitness

One of the biggest impediments to pursuing physical activity is time. When you, or both of you, have been used to freely exercising when you wanted and as long as you wanted, parenting can be a challenging adjustment. If you have two exercise schedules to juggle, it's even more challenging — but not impossible. Communicate, coordinate, and compromise.

For working parents this means examining the demands on your time and coming up with time slots where you can fit in exercise. Before work, during lunch or after work are possibilities. A run or bike ride before breakfast can easily be accomplished while the other person begins the morning routine. Shower facilities at your work place provide the option of cycling or running to work or on your lunch hour. Lunch hour workouts have the advantage of not cutting into time with your family. Fitness centers are another way to squeeze a workout into any of these time slots. Alternate times with your partner for variety. If your family is driving to a nearby destination, throw in a change of clothes in the car, strap on your running shoes and meet them there. Hire a sitter to come along if you are both competing in an event or take turns competing in different events. Look for races where you have friends or relatives nearby to watch your children. Early on, establish a reliable list of sitters for exercise scheduled on weekends.

It requires a bit more creativity if you're home with your child (or children). One mother of two pointed out that "not working outside the home allows more time flexibility but fewer child care options." Take turns with a relative, friend or neighbor watching each other's children. Consider starting a baby-sitting co-op or play group. A health club with child care facilities is a popular alternative. Seize the moments — no matter how brief! Work in a few abdominals, light weights, stretches or jumping rope while your children are involved with an activity. Kids love to join in and copy Mom. Running strollers, bike seats, trailers, and carriers allow you to exercise with your child. The moving motions of any of these pieces of equipment will soothe a cranky baby while you're enjoying the outdoors. Indoor exercise equipment allows you to get a workout during nap times or with your little one in a toy-filled playpen nearby.

Shelly, a single mother of two small children, tries to balance working full time, the demands of parenting and her desire to maintain her physical fitness. "I'm really forced to be clear about my priorities. I want to spend as much time as possible with my children and at the same time carve out time for some exercise. I think I am able to do this at the expense of social activities." Shelly tries to run during her lunch hour and uses a bike trailer for after work rides in good weather. A vigorous exercise video is an option after her children are settled for sleep. She emphasizes the need to balance exercise with a healthy diet and adequate rest.

Liz is also a single parent and works full time. During the first few months after her son was born, she used a NordicTrack™ to get back in shape before returning to Masters swim workouts. She hires a teen to watch her son during her twice weekly evening swims. She struggles with the emotional conflict of tagging on another sitting arrangement for her son but realizes the benefits she gains from swimming. For Liz, swimming provides her with a period of relaxed concentration. She feels revitalized and ready to engage in the demands of single parenting.

FIT FAMILIES

Many children today are in trouble due to lack of exercise. Risk factors for heart disease such as high cholesterol and obesity are being discovered in more and more children. According to the American Council on Exercise, as many as 40% of all children may have one of these risk factors (Gilliam, 1977).

What's the solution? Encourage physical activity in your children — the sooner, the better. Children who take up physical activities that are fun are healthier, have more self-confidence and self-esteem, a better body image, and a sense of how good it feels to be fit. It's these good feelings that will hopefully carry over into their adult lives as they maintain fitness through a healthy lifestyle.

The best way to get kids motivated and interested in exercise is to set a good example. You may be thinking that you are already being a good role model by running every day and training for your next marathon. Well, that's not enough. We need to participate in activities <u>with</u> our kids that are fun, like swimming, hiking, camping, and sledding, to name a few. Create opportunities for your child to get involved with community recreation programs, sports lessons, and summer camps. Provide the options but let your child choose what he or she <u>wants</u> to participate in . Support their efforts and offer praise along the way.

If you are a competitive athlete, it's important to emphasize your child's enjoyment and focus less on the "win" mentality. Kids will discover their own competitive drives in due time. What they need most is encouragement and praise for teamwork. They need to be supported as they handle their losses and failures. These are the skills that they will carry over into other areas of their adult lives, in relationships, jobs, and families. Provide children the opportunity to pursue activities they will enjoy when scholastic or collegiate sports are over, activities like hiking, skiing, cycling, or jogging. These and other sports help us return to the basic motivation for all exercise — the sheer pleasure of using our bodies.

A FATHER'S PERSPECTIVE

The other day I watched my 15 year old son wrestle in a high school tournament. He came to the match well prepared; he was conditioned, strong and determined — attributes essential to the sport. His participation in athletics goes back to his days as a toddler, when he began skiing, hiking, and canoeing with his parents. He sometimes rode along on his BMX bike while I ran or accompanied me to the weight room while I worked out. Later, when he joined youth soccer, I was the team's coach. He saw me compete in triathlons and cycle and foot races. Today our athletic interests, except for hiking, have diverged: his are scholastic team sports, mine are often solitary conditioning excursions. But we do share a mutual dedication to fitness. It's clear to me that his awareness, his commitment, and his self motivation were, to a large extent, generated through parental example and shared experiences.

PARENTS' PERSPECTIVES

Before we had our son, we both enjoyed a very active lifestyle: cross country skiing, hiking and backpacking, running, cycling, paddling canoes, and competing in road races. By doing these physical activities together — in fact, our first "date" was a bike ride — we created a strong bond. We wondered how things would change after having a child.

Father: From the very start, we included our son in our runs in a running stroller and later in cross country skiing outings in a back pack. The focus of my activities has changed. I don't compete as much as just participate. I still enjoy the same rewards of setting and achieving goals. These days, I get more gratification pushing a running stroller in a race than when, in the past, I used to cross the finish line ahead of others in my age group. The joy is greater because my son and I are sharing the pleasure of physical activity.

When he was almost two, I took him hiking up a mountain. It was only a twenty minute hike for an adult, but we took about an hour. I could tell by the look on his face and his little swagger as we broke out of the woods at the top, that he too was starting to sense the pleasure we all get from exerting ourselves and achieving a goal. I look forward to many experiences like these in the years ahead.

Mother: When our son was four weeks old, we hiked up a mountain carrying him in a front carrier. The view at the top was spectacular, but my eyes kept focusing on the small body sleeping in my arms. For me, parenthood has changed my views on a lot of things in life. Fitness is one example. Staying healthy and fit, and sometimes competitive, is important — but not as important as raising a healthy and happy child. Perhaps waiting until age 40 to start a family, working full time, and never having enough time, has helped me set priorities. Time moves quickly when it is measured by the rapid growth and development of your child.

As I watch our son grow and change, it becomes increasingly apparent that so much of what he learns is based on what he sees us, his parents, do. Just as pregnancy was an opportunity to maintain a balance between exercise, diet, and rest, raising a healthy child is an outgrowth of those same goals. I would like our son to enjoy the sheer fun of physical activity, whether it be recreational or sport-oriented. The rewards will provide him with self-confidence, self discipline, commitment, trust in his own body, and physical potential — all traits that will serve him well as he grows into an adult.

REFERENCE LIST

Agostini, R. (Ed). 1994. *Medical and orthopedic issues of active and athletic women*. Philadelphia: Hanley and Belfus, Inc.

American College of Obstetricians and Gynecologists. 1985. Technical Bulletin. *Exercise during pregnancy and the postnatal period*. Washington, D.C.

American College of Obstetricians and Gynecologists. 1994. Technical Bulletin. *Exercise during pregnancy and the postpartum period*. Washington, D.C.

Anderson, R. 1980. *Stretching*. Bolinas, Ca.: Shelter Publications.

Artal, R.; Rutherford, S.; Romen Y.; Kammula, R.K.; Dorey, F.J.; and Wiswell, R.A. 1986. Fetal heart rate responses to maternal exercise. *Am J Obstet Gynecol*. 155: 729-733.

Artal, R. 1992. Exercise and pregnancy. *Clin Spor Med*. April:11(2), 363-377.

Artal, R., and Subak-Sharpe, G.J. 1992. *Pregnancy and exercise*. New York: Delacorte Press.

Baechle, T., and Groves, B. 1992. *Weight training: Steps to success*. Champaign, Illinois: Leisure Press.

Bennet, J. 1993. *The weight training workbook*. Appleton, Wisconsin: JBBA Publishing.

Berga, S.L. 1993.How stress can affect ovarian function.
    Con Ob/Gyn. July: 87-94.

Berle, A.L. 1989. *Water aerobics*. Dubuque, Iowa: Kendall/Hunt
    Pub.Co.

Bicycling Magazine (Eds.). 1979. *Bicycling and your body*.
    Emmaus, Pa.: Rodale Press.

Borg, G.A. 1982. Psychophysical bases of perceived exertion. *Med Sci
    Sports Exerc*. 14:377-387.

Brems, M. 1984. *The fit swimmer: 120 workouts and training tips*.
    Chicago: Contemporary Books, Inc.

Carpenter, M.W.; Sady, S.P.; Hoegsberg, B.; Dady, M. A.; Haydon, B.;
    et al. 1988. Fetal response to maternal exertion.
    JAMA. 259: 3006-3009.

Clapp, J.F. 1985. Fetal heart rate response to running in mid-preg-
    nancy and late pregnancy. *Am J Obstet Gynecol*. 153: 251-252.

———. 1990. The course of labor after endurance exercise during
    pregnancy. *Am J Obstet Gynecol*. 163: 1799-1805.

Clapp, J.F., and Capeless, E.L. 1990. Neonatal morphometrics after
    endurance exercise during pregnancy.
    Am J Obstet Gynecol. 163: 1805-1811.

Clapp, J.F.; Little, K.D.; and Capeless, E.L. 1993. The fetal heart rate
    response to sustained recreational exercise.
    Am J Obstet Gynecol. 168: 198-206.
Clapp, J.F., and Little, K.D. 1995. Effect of recreational exercise on
    pregnancy weight gain and subcutaneous fat depostion. *Med Sci
    Sports Exerc*. 27(2): 170-177.

Cooper, K. 1982. *The aerobics program for total well-being*. New
    York: M. Evans and Co., Inc.

Cunningham, F.G.; MacDonald, P.; Gant, N.; Leveno, K.; and Gilstrap, L. 1993 *Williams Obstetrics, 19th Edition*. Norwalk, Conn.: Appleton and Lange.

Dale, B., & Roeber, J. 1982. *The pregnancy exercise book*. New York: Pantheon Books.

Davis, K. 1989. Pregnant & fit. *Women's Sports & Fitness*. Vol.11 (June): 50-55.

Dressendorfer, R.H., and Goodlin, R.C. 1980. Fetal heart rate response to maternal exercise testing. *Phys Sports Med*. 8: 91-94.

Edwards, M.J. 1986. Hyperthermia as a teratogen: a review of experimental studies and their clinical significance. *Teratogenesis Carcinog Mutagen*. 6: 563-582.

Eisenberg, A.; Murkoff, H.E.; and Hathaway, S.E. 1991. *What to expect when you're expecting*. New York: Workman Publishing.

Fishbein, E.G., and Phillips, M. 1990. How safe is exercise during pregnancy? *JOGNN*, 19(1): 45-49

Gilliam, T. 1977. Prevalence of coronary heart disease risk factors in active children 7-12 years of age. *Medicine & Science in Sports*. 9-21

Goldstein, R. (Ed). 1993. *Aerobics instructor manual*. Boston: American Council on Exercise and Reebok Univ. Press.

Gullion, L.. 1990. *The cross country primer*. New York: Lyons & Burford.

Hauth, J.O.; Gilstrap,L.C.; and Widmer, K. 1982. Fetal heart rate activity before and after maternal jogging during the third timester. *Am J Obstet Gynecol*. 142: 545-547.

Heed, P., and Mansfield, D. 1992. *Canoe racing*. Syracuse: Acorn Publishing.

Hetland, M.L.; Haarbo, J.; Christiansen, C.; and Larsen, T. 1993.
Running induces menstrual disturbances but bone mass is unaf-
fected, except in amenorrheic women.
Am J Med. Jul, 95(1):53-60.

Holstein, B. 1988. *Shaping up for a healthy pregnancy, instructor
guide.* Champaign, Illinois: Life Enhancement Publications.

Jarret, J.C., and Spellacy, W.N. 1983. Jogging during pregnancy: an
improved outcome? *Obstet Gynecol.* 61: 705-709.

Jarski, R.W., and Trippet, D.L. 1990. The risks and benefits of exercise
during pregnancy. *J Family Practice.* 30: 185-189.

Kelly, M., and Parsons, E. 1992. *The mother's almanac.*
New York: Doubleday.

Laskin, D. 1988. *Parents' book for new fathers.* New York: Ballantine
Books.

Lyndon, T. 1993. Swimming and pregnancy. *Swim.* 9(1):35-37.

Mansfield, D. 1988. *Skating on skis.* Syracuse: Acorn Publishing.

———. 1990. *Runner's guide to cross country skiing.* Syracuse:
Acorn Publishing.

Melpomene Institute for Women's Health Research. 1990. *The
bodywise woman.* Champaign, Illinois: Human Kinetics

McMurray, R.G.; Mottola, M.F.; Wolfe, L.A.; Artal,R.; Millar, L.; and
Pivarnik, J.M. 1993. Recent advances in understanding maternal
and fetal response to exercise.
Med Sci Sports Exer. 25(12): 1305-1321.

Mittelmark, R.A.; Wiswell, R.A.; and Drinkwater, B.L. 1991. *Exercise
in pregnancy.* Baltimore: Williams and Wilkins.

Naeye, R.L., and Peters, E.C. 1982. Working during pregnancy: effects
on the fetus. *Pediatrics.* 69: 724-727.

Otis, C.L. 1992. Exercise associated amenorrhea. *Clin Spor Med.* 11: 351. Rosen, L.W.; McKeag, D.B.; Hough, D.O.; et al. 1986. Pathogenic weight control behavior of female college athletes. *Phys Sports Med.* 14(1):79.

Rosen, L.W., and Hough, D.O. 1988. Pathogenic weight control behaviors of female college gymnasts. *Phys Sports Med.* 16(9): 141.

Shanan, J.; Brezinski, A.; Sulman, F.; et al. 1965. Active coping behavior, anxiety and corticol steroid excretion in the prediction of transient amenorrhea. *Behav Sci.* 10: 461.

Shangold, M., and Mirkin, G. (Eds). 1988 . *Women and exercise.* Philadelphia: FA Davis.

Shape Magazine. Spring 1994. Shape special guide to a fit pregnancy. Woodland Hills, Ca.

Sleamaker, R. 1989. *Serious training for serious athletes.* Champaign, Ilinois: Leisure Press.

Tafari, N.; Naeye, R.L.; and Gobezie, A. 1980. Effects of maternal undernutrition and heavy physical work during pregnancy on birth weight. *Br J Gynaecol.* 87: 222-226.

Verrilli, G.E., and Mueser, A.M. 1993. *While waiting.* New York: St. Martin's Press.

Weaver, S. 1991. *A woman's guide to cycling.* Berkeley: Ten Speed Press.

Whiteford, B. & Polden, M. 1984. *The postnatal exercise book: A six month fitness program for new mothers.* New York: Pantheon Books.

Webb, K.P.; Wolfe, L.A.; Hall, P.; Tranmer, J.E.; and McGrath, M.J. 1989. Fetal heart rate (FHR) responses to maternal exercise and physical conditioning (abstract). *Med Sci Sports Exerc.* 21:532.

RESOURCES

BOOKS

Bing, E. *Guide to Moving Through Pregnancy*. New York: Farrar, Straus and Giroux, 1992

Clark, N. *Nancy Clark's Sports Nutrition Guidebook*. Champaign, IL: Leisure Press, 1990

Erick, M. *No More Morning Sickness: A Survival Guide for Pregnant Women*. New York: Penguin Books, 1993

Eisenberg, A., Murkoff, H., Hathaway, S. *What to Eat When You're Expecting*. New York: Workman Publishing Co., Inc., 1986

Noble, E. *Essential Exercises For the Childbearing Years*, 3rd Edition

Olkin, S. K. *Positive Pregnancy Fitness*. Garden City, NJ: Avery. 1987

VIDEOTAPES

"The Expectant Father" Examines the father's perspective about pregnancy, childbirth and fatherhood. Available in local video stores or by calling (800) 745-1145

"Morning Sickness: All Day and All Night." Discusses relief measures and dietary advice for nausea in pregnancy.
To order, call (800) 540-6400

Exercise videos
Available at video stores or can be ordered through Collage Video which specializes in exercise videos. Call (800) 433-6769

Kathy Smith's Pregnancy Workout
Denise Austin's Pregnancy Plus Workout
Buns of Steel 8 - Pregnancy Workout
MomJam
Buns and Abs of Steel 9 - Post Pregnancy Workout

WORKOUT MUSIC

Sports Music, Inc. produces music tapes for all types of exercise (walking, stationary cycling, aerobics, etc.) (800) 878-4764 for a catalog.

CLOTHING

Workout wear or day wear for pregnancy Call the following numbers for a catalog.
Decent Exposures (206) 364-0488
A Pea in the Pod (800) 733-7373
Motherhood Maternity (800) 4MOM2BE
Motherwear, Inc. (800) 633-0303

Abdominal support wear
Bellybra by Basic Comfort, Inc.(800) 456-8687
The Prenatal Craddle Can be obtained by prescription through your health care provider and is usually covered by most
insurance. Call (800) 383-3068
Reenie Maternity Belt (800) 321-4804

EQUIPMENT
The following prices are approximate and may vary. Most of this equipment is available in sporting good stores or by catalog.

Baby Carriers
Kid Carrier by Tough Traveler ($137)
Panda Child Carrier by Kelty, Inc. ($115)
Ultra Kiddie Pack by Gerry ($60)

Bike Trailers
Burley Design Cooperative ($365)
Winchester Originals, Inc. ($350)

Pulk - children's sled for pulling while cross country skiing.
Available at nordic ski shops.
Mountainsmith ($389)

Running strollers
Huffy Ride "N" Run - a bike trailer and running stroller ($229)
Huffy Double Gerry Rollerbaby - for two children ($249)
Racing Strollers, Inc. Available in single and double and single models.
($209)-324) Call (800) 241-1848
Weebok's Multi-Baby Stroller ($289) Call (800) 541-7064

ORGANIZATIONS

American College of
Nurse-Midwives
818 Connecticut Ave., NW Suite 900
Washington, D.C. 20006

American College of Obstetricians
 and Gynecologists
409 12th Street, SW
Washington, D.C. 20024

American College of Sports Medicine
401 West Michigan Street
Indianapolis, Indiana 46202

American Council on Exercise
5820 Oberlin Drive, Suite 102
San Diego, Ca. 92121

National Strength and
Conditioning Association
PO Box 38909
Colorado Springs, Co. 80937

Help and support during pregnancy and after:

Depression After Delivery
PO Box 1282 Morrisville, Pa. 19067

La Leche League - a national support group with local chapters
which provides information on breastfeeding. (800) LA LECHE

Postpartum Education Hotline 1-(805) 564-3888

Sidelines National Support Network -a support group for women
who are bedridden during pregnancy.
PO Box 1808 Laguna Beach, Ca. 92652   (714) 497-2265

Index